PRAISE FOR
THE HEALER IS WITHIN

"Katherine has written a heartfelt, inspirational, and insightful weaving of her personal story with insights and invitations for the reader to drop into direct experience of their own deep capacity for self-transformation and healing."

Carrie Lafferty, PT, Guild Certified Feldenkrais
Practitioner, Master QI Gong Teacher

"*The Healer is Within* is an energizing and inspiring read. With tremendous authenticity and humor, Katherine Hand shares her own healing journey, seamlessly interwoven with springboards to help you develop your own. She understands all too well the pressure that many of us feel to prioritize achievement above connecting with our bodies, our intuition, and our spiritual needs, and she gently guides readers towards more fulfilling ways to live."

Rachel Goldsmith Turow, Ph.D., Author of
*Mindfulness Skills for Trauma and PTSD:
Practices for Recovery and Resilience*

"*The Healer is Within* includes so many valuable nuggets of wisdom and offers hope, useful tools and references, and a path to healing for anyone struggling through life challenges, big or small. It's a terrific book to read if you're looking to find your own inner source of strength, knowledge, resilience and growth."

Elisa Mandell Keller, Principal, EMK Strategic Consulting

"*The Healer is Within* is a courageous story of a woman who transmutes her truth into wisdom in a deeply vulnerable yet inspiring way."

Johanna Rabin, HeartRising Coach,
Biodynamic Cranial Sacral Therapist

THE
HEALER
IS
WITHIN

THE HEALER IS WITHIN

A Healing Memoir and Transformational Guide

KATHERINE HAND

Published by Katherine Hand, Seattle, WA

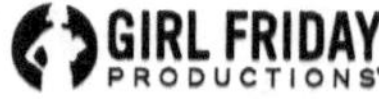

Designed by Girl Friday Productions
www.girlfridayproductions.com

Edited by Anna Katz
Image credits: cover © Shutterstock/Sergey
Nivens, Shutterstock/ BAIVECTOR

ISBN (paperback): 9798663243988

First edition

Printed in the United States of America

To my family, friends, spiritual teachers and healing guides. Thank you and I love you.

CONTENTS

ACKNOWLEDGEMENTS

Deepest Gratitude to: Carolyn Marquardt, Arran Franklin, David Handsome, Henry Lu, Carrie Lafferty, Rachel Turow, Llewellyn Packia Raj, Kent Moberly Ellen McCown, Susanna Marie, Bill and Patricia Clum, Craig Matsu Pissot, Elisa Mandell, Johanna Rabin, Anna Katz, Joanna Wardisko, Corey Fagan, Carrie Kincaid Elaine Mowery, Shehreen Johnson, Victoria Erickson, Katherine MacKenett, my sanga friends near and far, my family and my creative tribe.

INTRODUCTION

As a highly empathic and sensitive child, I couldn't stand to see anyone suffer. In grade school, whenever a kid got their feelings hurt, I'd come rushing in to take them on a "wisdom-walk" during which we'd hash out the injustices and emotional woundings inherent to life on the playground. In hindsight, this is when I began my career as a healer.

Later in life, I answered my soul's calling more formally by becoming a psychotherapist, running therapy groups for the better part of ten years. This experience was highly rewarding and allowed allowing me the privilege of witnessing many people's healing journeys. Through this process, I developed a keen interest in the concept of neuroplasticity, or the ability to rewire the brain. I eventually transitioned into a neuroscience research role and began working on a large-scale research study that investigated how we could improve the lives of those who suffered from chronic pain. It was while working on that study that I was injured in a way that would change my life forever.

Because of that experience, I had to reassess what it means to be a healer. I like to be in charge of things, and I was much more comfortable coming to others' aid than asking for aid for myself. During my long recovery, I had to let go of the identity of someone who helps the healing process of others and accept a new identity of someone who desperately needed help and, at the same, had the power within to heal herself.

Though I might have felt like it in my darkest moments, I was not alone.

We are all healing in some form or another. I'm not sure I've ever met anyone who wasn't in the process of healing, whether they recognized it as such or not. Any kind of striving to change one's circumstances is an attempt at healing, a creative impulse much like a plant turning toward the sun. Yet often, when we've suffered greatly, we have a tendency to look outside of ourselves for someone who will "heal" us, to find a savior who will save us from our suffering. This can manifest in benign ways, like looking to that physical therapist or AA sponsor to help us strengthen our bodies or our resolve. It can lean toward the unhealthy, like when we jump from diet to diet in the hopes that the next one will be *the* one that not just helps alleviate hypertension but gets us closer to some untenable ideal. And, sometimes, it can be downright detrimental, like when we attach ourselves to a charismatic religious leader who takes cash or check and does not genuinely have our best interests at heart.

We all need guides to help us along our healing journeys. But what each of us who are seeking have in common is that the journey requires us to claim our personal power, to tap into the innate healing wisdom within. You are the one who must decide what's right for you—though the care and advice of doctors, therapists, alternative healers, spiritual teachers, a significant other, family, and friends are essential in supporting your journey, at the end of the day, it's up to you to make tough choices as you work toward health and healing. You are the only one who can truly heal yourself.

As a healer, and as someone who's undertaken her own long healing process, I am here to offer you the wisdom I've gained along the way, wisdom that I hope will propel you forward on your journey. My most sincere hope is that you find inspiration, wisdom, empowerment, and a sense of connection, knowing that you're not alone.

CHAPTER 1

Divine Whispers

*"You are not going with the flow, you are the
flow. Creating that stream and current with
every step, intention and breath."*

—*Victoria Erickson*

In 2016, I was in the middle of an incredible transition. A long-term relationship was coming to a drawn-out, painful close, and I was packing up my former life in a nice little house near Lincoln Park in West Seattle to move into a new apartment complex alone above Puget Sound.

While trying to heal from my personal heartbreak, I was doing my best to make a contribution to the world, to live an inspired life and to work to alleviate suffering in whatever capacity I could. I had made some career shifts from working with children as a psychotherapist to a job in neuroscience research through the University of Washington School of

Medicine. Located at a local hospital nearby, we were studying those who lived with varying degrees of chronic pain, many as a result of spinal cord injuries, in what was one of the largest clinical trials to date.

I'd often go walking with my dear friend Amanda along Alki, a stretch of sidewalk alongside the shore right below my new place. With her I could process the myriad of changes in my life, and she confided in me about her eight-year-long recovery after a horrific rock-climbing fall and then, soon thereafter, getting in a car accident. Her injury had not just derailed but essentially taken over her life, and yet she moved through the pain, grief, and frustration with admirable grace and dignity.

I too had been going through my own recovery process, after falling down a rain-soaked stairway while knocking on doors for the 2012 election. Since then I'd been seeing an alternative medical practitioner, who had managed to alleviate the terrible concussion I'd sustained when the doctors and nurses in the ER had basically told me to wait and see and hope for the best. She told me that she was the *only* one who could help me, and though I felt uncertain about her claim, I'd spent $250 per session, going several times a month for four years afraid of the consequences if it turned out she was right.

Amanda was like an angel sent from above, a steadying presence in my rocking boat of a life. I was heartbroken about all that I'd lost yet excited about the possibilities that my new situation might bring. On those days when she and I didn't meet, I'd wake up early and go out for a morning run. There's no better way to start the day than moving through the quiet of morning before the noise of traffic and garbage trucks and other humans rushing into their days, with only the sounds of water lapping at the beach and a murder of crows squawking over their breakfast. Life was beginning to take a beautiful twist, and I was beginning to feel like I was in the flow.

The only hitch in my stride occurred when I came back from my run to encounter one of my neighbors struggling to get in his car from his wheelchair. Not wanting to be rude, I'd say hello then continue on my way, but often I'd look out my apartment window to see him still at it. It took him about ten minutes to complete a task that took me less than 20 seconds. I felt a mix of empathy and inspiration, and it made me realize how much I took for granted as an able-bodied person. Each time I encountered him, I'd think to myself, *I couldn't live without the use of my legs. I'm such an active and athletic person, I don't think I could go on if I lost the ability to walk.*

After a quick shower and a cup of coffee, I'd head off to work. I was always excited about what the day would bring, what kind of new discoveries my fellow team members and I would make. Their enthusiasm for the work and determination to help the participants matched my own, but like most research projects, our study was underfunded, and we were generally overworked. In my experience, people in the research field tend to be driven by altruism, and most of us end up putting work before self. Ours was a team of six, but we were doing the work of about twenty people. "We need to hire more people," I'd tell my bosses. "We can afford to hire three more people. We're confident you can handle the rest," they'd say.

So that's what I did: I handled it. I worked and worked and worked and worked. And I was proud of what we were doing, how we were trying to better understand chronic pain and figure out better practices for easing it. But my unwavering passion for the project clouded my survival instincts, leading me into the trifecta of stress, anxiety, and sleeplessness that would be my undoing. Soon, instead of hopping out of bed in the morning, I began to wake up with a feeling of dread in the pit of my stomach. What new aggravation would the day bring? How many fires would there be to put out? How was I going to fit forty hours of work into an eight-hour day? I'd become completely tapped out with nothing left to give it or anyone.

I was at least aware enough to spot a breaking point on the horizon, and so toward the middle of September I asked my boss for a day off. One single day. *That should get me back on track,* I thought. I'd sleep in, do a load of laundry or two, maybe read a novel in the bath, then return to work right as rain. My boss approved my request, and at the end of the workday before my day off, she called out to me as I gathered up my phone and keys. "Read this," she said simply, handing me a book by Dr. David Hanscom called *Back in Control: A Spine Surgeon's Roadmap Out of Chronic Pain.*

At home, I tossed the book on my two-foot pile of unopened mail, half completed paperwork, and all the various bits and bobs that were part of my never-ending to-do list. Then I promptly forgot about it.

The morning of my sacred, much-needed day off was beautiful and sunny, not too hot, one of those perfect late summer days in Seattle. I took to that strip of beach by my apartment, strolling along unrushed and the most peaceful I'd been since I couldn't remember how long. Alone with my own thoughts, I could admit that I wanted off the career treadmill. The life I'd envisioned, in which I would write books, give TED talks, and, for one day a week, work as a psychotherapist, all the while getting enough sleep, veggies, and downtime, seemed as far away as Never Never Land. But I wasn't ready to give up just yet. *Please,* I asked the universe, *put me in a place where I don't have to work on that stressful research project. Please put me in a place that will allow me to carry out my soul work.*

Be careful what you wish for.

About a week later, I saw my alternative medical practitioner who was also clairvoyant. During our treatment, she told me that I was going to get "really slowed down."

"Be careful," she said. It was an ominous yet vague warning. I had no idea what she was talking about, yet I had a visceral reaction; a feeling in my bones that something was about to go down.

Two days later, on September 26, 2016, I went out for my morning jog as usual. Generally I used this occasion to problem solve in my head, and now I needed to do so more than ever because later that morning, we would be kicking off the first day of a large-scale clinical trial. Our brilliantly crafted, complex study design had landed us an enormous grant, and everything was riding on our ability to prove that we deserved it, that we would hit real milestones in our mission to save thousands of people suffering from chronic pain.

At first, something felt . . . off. Then, as I was fanaticizing about how the day would unfold, I began to feel pain pulsating throughout my right hip. It burned and throbbed, spreading from this central locus to my low back and then into every cell of my body.

I became paralyzed in a matter of minutes, falling to my knees in the sand. I tried to take a breath but couldn't. My body was no longer my body; it was a strobe of pain, flashing and flashing and flashing.

You would think that in this moment, when I was paralyzed with pain, I would sit still, pull out my cell phone, and call a friend for help. That is not what I did. Instead I thought, *Shit I'm going to be late for work.*

Somehow I got to my feet and over the course of an hour and a half, during which I worried more about my tardiness than my health, I managed to crawl/drag myself the mile or so back home. People stopped and stared. Every time I fell, someone would stop and ask me if I needed a hand up or offered the use of their cell phone. "I'm fine," I'd say and keep going.

In this state I went to work. *I'll go to the doctor at the end of the day,* I told myself.

I can't remember how I got through that day, but I did. In fact, it's hard for me to remember much about the following days, weeks, and months, during which I visited the emergency room countless times. My hip had dislocated, throwing my pelvis into a forward rotation that pinched nerves and created a ripple of locked muscles up through my thoracic spine. Once the initial adrenaline of the injury had worn off, pain completely colonized my awareness, and so now the actual events of that time are a blur. I know I saw a variety of specialists who had no idea what was wrong or how to relieve my pain. Every time I explained to a doctor what had happened and what I was experiencing, they looked worried in a way that indicated both concern for me and confusion about what to do. They put forward all kinds of diagnoses from multiple sclerosis to stroke, Lou Gehrig's Disease to paralysis of unknown origin. Over the course of the following months, I obtained crutches, a leg cart, and a wheelchair, along with many other devices to help me move. But my declining mobility wasn't the worst part; the worst part was the unrelenting pain. It was pain so severe that the strongest narcotic drugs couldn't touch it.

If you've ever been in pain, you know that there really are no words to describe it. All I can say is that suddenly and unexpectedly that which I had been studying from a scientific distance was upon me, within me, a chronic, unceasing pain, like being boiled alive. It did not leave me for even one second, and I couldn't move or eat or sleep, let alone work on the project that had given my life so much meaning. Every doctor's appointment brought more worried looks but no answers and certainly no relief. I fell into a deep despair and kept falling, falling, down into a chasm of helplessness and hopelessness, with no rock bottom in sight.

Consumed by the darkness, I decided to end it.

DIVINE WHISPERS

The divine is always communicating with us just as we are communicating with the divine, in a continuous flow of dialogue unfolding at all times. More often than not, it tends to manifest in subtle whispers, coincidences, and serendipities. Recognizing it requires that we get quiet and truly listen, that we allow ourselves to be open and available. And it means that we should be aware of what we say on our side of the conversation.

Easier said than done, especially when stress and anxiety jam up the radar. Pain, whether physical or psychic, can make us feel like we are alone in the universe, that the pain is the only thing that exists, that matters. It can be so loud that nothing else can get through, so huge it's all we can see, so all-consuming. This is where I found myself in the months after what seemed to be a spontaneous back injury. All I could hear was my pain—that is why I was desperate for escape. I felt like there was no other way out.

But what if I had been listening to the little whispers and seeing the serendipities long before that terrible moment on the beach? They certainly existed, only I was too caught up in my cycle of stress and more stress to pay attention. And so I had to go through hell before I started noticing how the divine unfolds. In retrospect, I can see three important messages that I had ignored:

> Message 1: My friend Amanda telling me about her eight year long journey to heal a massive trauma, and her showing me that it's possible to face pain with grace and dignity.

> Message 2: Watching my neighbor move himself from wheelchair to car and thinking, over

and over again, *I could never do that.* Perhaps
the universe took this as a dare. It might have
thought to itself, *Oh yeah? Let's find out.*

Message 3: My boss handing me a book about
spinal pain and healing on my way out the
door.

Message 4: My being involved in a study of
chronic pain.

Frequently, we see the signs after the damage has been done.
How often during an illness have you looked back on the previous days or weeks and recognized a nascent symptom for what
it was? Perhaps it was directly linked to your current situation—
an ache in the knee that you ignored, someone sneezing on
you on the subway. Perhaps it wasn't quite so obvious in the
moment. A book about spinal injury is just a book about spinal
injury—that is, until you yourself have a spinal injury. That's
one of those hints it's hard to see at the time but in retrospect
the message is clear.

Then there are those who are able to read the writing on
the wall ahead of time. Some call this "intuition"—a person
has a feeling in the pit of her stomach that tells her not to go
to work in the Twin Towers on a crisp late summer day in
2001. Or, more prosaically, a person feels a tickle in the back
of his throat that compels him to cancel his happy hour plans
and instead go home and drink some lemon ginger tea and
hit the hay early, thus nipping that oncoming cold in the bud.
Sometimes people think of it as a kind of outside intervention,
like when Pittsburgh steel baron Henry Clay Frick, for example, canceled his trip on the *Titanic* because his wife sprained
her ankle.[1] Was that a coincidence? Sure. Was it divine intervention? Absolutely.

It's a cliché to say that higher intelligence works in mysterious ways, which just goes to show that it's true. So how can you become more astute at catching on to the clues? We'll talk more about this in chapter 3, but for now I'll say that it's about what you pay attention to. This is the basic premise of cognitive behavior therapy—the way you think impacts your life and vice versa. If you assume that everyone is out to get you, you are more likely to see signs of manipulation and maltreatment and, in turn, behave in ways that are guarded or even shifty. This will then illicit guarded or shifty behaviors from others; a cycle that serves to reinforce that original belief. If, on the other hand, you believe that humans are mostly generous and good, then you will notice friendliness more readily, snark will roll off your back, and you yourself will behave in generous ways that invite reciprocity. The same goes for health and healing. If you recognize that your energy is much lower than it was last month, and you're having trouble remembering simple things, and you have started to get headaches every evening, then you might do something about it before it turns dire. Instead, if you are too focused on other things—work, childcare, student loans—to notice the signs of mounting exhaustion, you are likely to wait until it has snowballed into a full-blown illness or injury before doing anything about it. It all depends on what you are paying attention to. In that sense, illness, injury, and trauma are divine interventions and invitations to wake up. This is their first gift.

A GIFT IN UNUSUAL WRAPPING

No one wants to suffer or asks to suffer or deserves to suffer. Like wealth, illness, injury, and trauma are unevenly distributed. Those born into privilege versus poverty owe as much to Lady Luck as do those who get hurt versus those who somehow manage to mostly avoid life's scratches and stumbles. (Of course, no matter how rich or healthy a person is, life always has the final word.) We don't consciously choose illness, injury, the difficulties that find us, or even the difficulties that we create. What we do on a daily basis for self and community care, and what we do when confronted with hardship—that is where our choices lie.

When you ignore divine whispers for a long time, louder and louder ones will come along until they finally get your undivided attention. I for one would have much rather received a concise memo informing me that I was burning myself out, and that I needed to take a real break. Not that I would have taken it seriously, hence the excruciating back pain. This is the first gift of illness, injury, or trauma: it forces us to pause and to take ourselves and our lives seriously. An unfortunate event can be read like a bright neon sign telling you that there's something in your life you have neglected. Or it can be read like a wake-up call, a blaring alarm, a slap in the face. It is a shout from the divine that won't be ignored.

What your condition is trying to tell you is that the choices you made before clearly no longer work—in fact, it is those very choices that have led you astray, and now the illness or injury steps in to assist you in getting your life back on track, or conscientiously coming up with a new track altogether. Old habits die hard—sometimes illness and injury act as mercenaries, doing the tough job of killing them.

Sometimes a migraine is just a migraine, but then again if you look deeper, you might discover that there's more to it. A short-term illness like a cold or the flu might force you to pay attention to your fluid intake and increase your amount of rest time. Becoming injured in a profound way such as tearing your ACL might force you to stop skiing and start creating more balance in your body through physical therapy; being diagnosed with a debilitating disease like Crohn's might force you to assess your diet and the ways in which you manage inflammation. On a deeper level, in these three scenarios the body halts life, forcing you to reassess and rearrange your priorities. (Which, after a little while, you might forget and then have to be reminded by going through the whole rigamarole again.) In the most extreme cases, it might involve coming to term with one's own death and figuring out how to live the best life possible with the time remaining.

Whatever the particulars of your condition, its gift is that it signals some kind of misalignment that needs to be redressed. Perhaps it is misalignment with your highest purpose, and now you must look deeply at yourself and your life, and make changes that you otherwise wouldn't.

Therefore, from a spiritual perspective, illness can be viewed as a step toward wholeness. There is a profound intelligence within your experience, a higher lesson to be learned, a purpose to revealed and wisdom to be gained.

REFUSING THE GIFT

Over the course of my recovery, I've met a countless number cancer survivors at various healing retreats who have claimed that their disease was the greatest blessing they'd ever received because it forced them to completely transform their lives. A reminder of one's mortality is great motivation for reshuffling priorities and pursuing new paths; for doing all those things we want to do but hadn't quite worked up the nerve to do and for shaking off the status quo and seeking profound fulfillment. Cancer is one of many diseases that give people the permission to make different choices that they wouldn't have given themselves otherwise.

Now, I am not suggesting that most people get a cancer diagnosis on Tuesday and then start posting #blessed on

Instagram on Wednesday. The more common, and, perhaps rational reaction is to want to push it away. The ego, that little voice that tells you that you are separate from the rest of the universe, has a few key ways it likes to trick you into making a difficult situation worse. These are:

Denial

Everything is A-OK, we say to ourselves, even when all signs point to the contrary. We pretend like nothing's wrong and go about our day, even when our bodies or intuitions are begging us to do otherwise. For weeks my friend Flor lived with a cough that grew more and more terrible by the hour. She hacked and hacked all day in her office, while walking to her car, while she cooked dinner. Her cough kept her up all night, and it kept her husband up too until finally, he lost his patience and took her to the hospital, where the doctors diagnosed her with pneumonia and then drained a quart of murky brown fluid from her lung. It took that and a week's stay in the hospital for her to get the message. Denial was my preferred method of health management too, but, as I discovered the hard way, that only works for so long.

Judgment and Blame

No one wants cancer. No one wants ingrown toenails or parking tickets either. But that's life. It just is. These things happen and will continue to happen forever and ever, not just to you but to everybody. But the ego wants to put a value judgment on it. Cancer is bad. Ingrown toenails are bad. Traffic tickets are bad. Can you feel what happens in your body when you read that, when you associate the word "bad" with reality? For me, it's a constriction; a tensing. It makes me want to flee or fight, not deal.

A few years ago, my friend Aimee needed to take a week off for an operation to remove an ovarian cyst. In the spirit of transparency—and to disrupt the conditioning that told her she should be ashamed of her "lady problems"—she told her coworkers the reason for her paid time off. "But you do yoga," one coworker said. "And you eat well, don't you? You don't smoke, do you? Drink conventional milk?" And so on and so on.

It's one thing for Aimee to do an honest and loving self-assessment of her lifestyle when faced with health problems; it's quite another for a coworker to interrogate her to try to pinpoint Aimee's "mistake." In essence, he was taking on the role of the ego in blaming her for her affliction.

For me and many others, that internal judgment and blame of the ego is the most difficult to deal with; more difficult than the judgment and blame of others. When I first got injured, I spent a lot of time asking what I had done to deserve this health crisis. *This illness/injury/trauma is bad*, that internal judge/ego tells us, *and since you have it, you must be bad too. You must have done something bad to have brought this on yourself. It is your fault.* Now how is that supposed to help?

Control

At this point, you may be thinking: *This di-sease is bad, and it's my fault, so now I'm going to fight it with every weapon at my disposal. I will only eat kale. I will never stay up later than 8:00 p.m. I will cancel all people whom I don't get along with absolutely perfectly. I will meditate two hours every day. I will do everything right from now on.*

How long do you think this new plan will last? I can tell you: not very. You will never be able to control every aspect of your life and even if you could, you are likely still going to get hurt or sick. Plus, this tamping down is another way to avoid the message—if you're so busy micro-managing every detail of your life, then you are not paying attention to the big picture.

Victimization

The flip side of the control trap is the victim trap. *This disease is bad. It's my fault. I'm therefore a terrible person and too weak or stupid to change things.* Cue the violins.

You may not feel ready or willing to make the changes that illness or your spiritual self is propelling you to make. That's fair—change is really hard. But the problem lies in the snowballing: helplessness ensues, lifestyle choices remain unchanged, and the problem stagnates or gets worse. You start to *resign* yourself—which is wholly different than *accepting*—to your pain and the increasing limitations it creates in your life. Every time you give away your personal power, it is replaced by equal measure helplessness, and so you spiral down.

RECEIVING THE GIFT

Taking responsibility is not the same as blaming, controlling, or feeling like a victim. Remember that phrase "Shit happens"? There's a reason it caught on like wildfire in the early 1980s— what a relief! Shit just happens. Your condition isn't a punishment or a curse. It's a tool, a launching point, a revelation of hidden aspects of yourself that need integrating. It's a blessing or maybe even a gift. Now you can begin to relax into the situation and, ideally, take a deeper look at what's going on below the surface.

The more you can lean into the flow of change that illness brings about, the more healing you will generate in your life. Allowing the gift of your condition to manifest enables you to move towards greater health and vitality. Now is the time to focus on realigning yourself with your highest good and pursuing your deeper purpose. As you begin to truly listen to the intelligence within your condition, you'll become empowered to take informed action.

> *When we truly examine what illness forces us*
> *to change, we can see that these changes are*
> *always supporting our highest good.*

True healing involves addressing all aspects of yourself, in particular those that make you uncomfortable, especially if you've been living with chronic health conditions. That sticking point, the point where we'd rather pick up our phones or turn on the T.V. or do anything other than continue a certain line of questioning . . . that's where the good stuff is. Are you in a soul-sucking job? Is your nervous system in a permanent state of fight-or-flight? Are you in an unhealthy intimate relationship or marriage?

I don't want to paint with a broad brush or imply that I know you, your life, or any answers. For some people, the stress of a corporate job is well worth the paycheck. Lord knows we all have compelling reasons for keeping that overly critical parent or passive-aggressive partner around. The last thing I want to do is shame someone for not getting an optimal amount of exercise or eating enough kale when they have three kids, a full-time job, an ailing spouse, an ancient washing machine, and a stack of bills to deal with. There is no one-size-fits-all. (I wish!) Rather, it's about each person being able to assess their own life and make wiggle room for new priorities. It's about taking responsibility where possible to create the conditions for healing that are right for them in that moment.

I'd like to invite you to take a deep breath and consider your symptoms. Think about any diagnosis you've either been given or that you have given yourself. Answer the following questions as honestly as possible.

Reflection Questions

- Looking back, can you pinpoint signs of dis-ease that you ignored? Serendipities, coincidences, intuitions, divine whispers?
- What is the symptom or symptoms of your condition that most powerfully grab your attention?
- What is your initial reaction to pain or discomfort? Do you tend to deny, fight, control, judge, blame, feel victimized?
- What do you think your condition is meant to teach you? What lessons are you resisting?
- What positive changes have you made in your life due to your condition?
- What are the new patterns, priorities and possibilities that have emerged as a result of your condition?
- Are there positive changes you know you should make but are resisting? If so, why?
- What do you need to change in your life to truly heal?
- What are the gifts of your condition?

CHAPTER 2

The Alchemy of Surrender

*"Transformation is what happens on the other
side of surrender."*

—*Unknown*

It had been three months since I'd dragged myself along Alki, three months of sleepless nights, of being unable to get out of bed, of days spent crying, of visiting the ER only to be sent home with another impotent prescription. On TV and online Santa Claus was selling beer and cars and occasionally toys for kids. Outside my window was an expanse of gray water dotted with rain which I watched from my apartment as I lay in bed or on the couch consumed by pain.

As the days got shorter, I finally had a reason to be hopeful. After running into dead end after dead end, I'd found an amazing physical therapist who'd put me in touch with a few new specialists, who seemed to be circling closer to the cause of my injury and effective treatment. After three months of growing despair, I was now catching glimpses of a future without relentless agony. Those glimpses were my only lifeline, and I held on for dear life.

But just as change seemed within reach, everyone went on Christmas vacation. I've since heard the same story many times from others who were in desperate need and left to their own devices at the end of the year while doctors and nurses and other medical professionals go on their much-deserved holidays. At the time I didn't realize this was a common problem. Rather, I felt completely alone with my pain in what is supposed to be the most wonderful time of the year, and suddenly suicide seemed like the only way out.

The thing is, before my involvement in the chronic pain research study, I would never have considered suicide as an option. I loved life, even with its downs and disappointments. But that was before my own experience with chronic pain. Now I'd tried every drug under the sun, every muscle relaxant and opioid, few of which gave me even a minute of relief, and those that did made it worse once they wore off. Now I'd felt the hopelessness firsthand. Now I understood why someone would choose death over a life lived in pain.

And so I devised a foolproof plan and carried it out.

I adjusted the bedcovers, closed my eyes, and in a moment knew I was leaving this world. "Now I lay me down to sleep, I pray the lord my soul to keep," I whispered. "If I should die before I wake, I pray the lord my soul to . . . " Before I could finish, I was transported into a dark tunnel. The Buddhists call this the "bardo," a transitional realm where one's soul goes between death and rebirth. I saw no welcoming light. I saw no towering gates to heaven. I was trapped in an endless tunnel of darkness traveling at the speed of light.

Twenty hours later, my body jolted awake like I'd been shocked with a defibrillator. I sat upright in bed with a gasp and in an instant, I came back to this world. Immediately I knew that I wasn't the same person who'd tried to leave life behind. In the abyss, the bardo, I'd remembered who I was and why I was here. as myself in this life. Enveloped by a surging power, I sensed myself moving into a place of deep transformation.

I lay there just breathing, feeling myself letting go. Letting go of the life I'd been chasing, a life of striving for prestigious job titles, of trying to bolster my intimate partners while completely ignoring myself, of numbing discomfort with food and "busyness," of always wanting more and no matter how much I got, always feeling empty. What I learned in those key moments was that I would never be fulfilled in that life, that I would never find truth if I stayed tethered to conventional social values and pressures, or to the person I had been. I was so clearly walking away from the very life that kept me disconnected from the truth. Ahead of me was a murky course toward an unknown, yet I had a new clarity, strength, and power that would lead me forward.

Not that I was happy about it. In fact, I was fucking pissed to be here; to be alive in my earthly state. There was a jumble of other swirling emotions, but that was the primary one: anger. After all that, and here I was, lying in my bed, as alive and hurting as I'd ever been. I went over the plan in my mind, looking for miscalculations and mistakes. *My plan was flawless.* I concluded. *What the hell?*

After a few minutes of helpless fury, I reached over to the bedside table, picked up my phone, and turned it on. It came to life and I scrolled down to the number of my best friend, Sarah. I cleared my very dry throat as the phone rang.

"Kat?" Sarah said.

"I . . . I tried to kill myself," I rasped. "Can you come over?"

There was a moment of silence before she answered. "Of course. I'm in the line at the grocery store, almost done paying. Be there in a sec."

I must have passed out, because all of a sudden the sound of knocking woke me. The knocking turned into banging as I painfully shifted over to the edge of the bed and placed my feet on the floor. The banging turned into pounding, the sound ricocheting through my head like a 747 clearing the runway as I made my way to the door.

There, in the hallway, stood Sarah with two full grocery bags.

"Hello," she said, remaining eerily calm while strolling past me into my kitchen. "Well," she went on, looking everywhere but at me, "before I take you to the hospital, I better get these groceries in the fridge so they don't go bad."

"OK, sure," I said. As if we had all the time in the world, we leisurely reorganized my refrigerator, consolidating her new items with mine. Pushing my 2 percent milk to the side, she said, "You know, you really need to buy organic. And is that conventional lettuce? You're basically eating a pesticide salad." Then she stopped, her hand on the door handle.

"I promise to eat only organic foods from now on," I said. Here I was, reluctantly awake from a self-induced coma, and I was talking about organics? I almost laughed. I almost cried. Slowly, Sarah turned to look at me. In her eyes was a reflection of my own terror. Just like that, our denial vanished, and reality hit us like a ton of bricks. "C'mon," she said, "let's go."

We didn't talk much on the way to the hospital. "Why didn't you call me before . . . ?" Sarah asked at one point, not quite finishing the sentence.

"There was nothing anyone could do," I said.

She dropped me off at the emergency room entrance, then went to park. A nurse approached with a wheelchair, which I gratefully sat in to be wheeled into the waiting room. I didn't have to wait long—once I'd written the big bad S-word on the intake form, a nurse ushered me into a private room, where she and some other nurses and doctors gathered my story and took my vitals. I could read the shock on their faces; how was I even breathing, let alone standing there before them, telling them what I had done?

After waiting a few hours for test results to come back, my doctor shuffled in to deliver some news. He cleared his throat. "Um, there is no medical explanation as to why you are still alive." He kept his eyes down on his clipboard. "But here you are.

DOING EVERYTHING RIGHT

Most of us come to believe that if we do everything right, everything will be alright. If we attain certain standards in our lives—landing the dream job, buying the house with the big windows and the view of the lake, reducing to an 18.5 BMI, marrying that perfect someone—then we will be happy and free. For us, Nirvana is located here on earth, and we're always *almost* there. It's just down the street, right around the next corner, and we'll arrive just as soon as we achieve that next big milestone. So what if it takes sixty-, seventy-, even eighty-hour workweeks, straining to get that perfect photo to post on social media, always striving for the future and never really experiencing the present?

We're conditioned to force, to control, to "make things happen," all too often pushing away the very peace we truly desire. We unintentionally choose suffering over serenity, never questioning whose expectations we are trying to meet. But the reality is that most of us can't sustain the fast-paced, competitive, achievement-driven, high-tech, isolated lifestyle to which we've become addicted. It eventually becomes impossible to stay so tightly bound to societal expectations while juggling more than we can handle while also going to extreme measures to put on the facade that "everything is all right."

No wonder so many of us end up relying on a combination of antidepressants, the upper of coffee in the morning and the downer of alcohol at night, the fat-and-sugar hit of fast food, and the pseudo-connection of the Internet to numb us out and get us through. No wonder we drown ourselves in debt trying to keep up with the Joneses, why we look to new cars and designer jeans for validation, why we put off our dreams until we can check off everything on our to-do list. We walk through life with our eyes shut tight, moving further and further from the truth . . . until we reach our tipping point.

This is where I'd found myself on that late September day when I'd decided to take my own life. I had achieved so much, and yet I felt empty. I'd worked and worked and worked and yet never felt satisfied, let alone finished. I'd done everything "right" and yet my own body had betrayed me. The world had reneged on our agreement that I would work and push and strive nonstop and in return, it would give me an insta-perfect life, a white picket fence, a sense of peace. So I got angry.

THE INVERSION OF ANGER: VICTIMHOOD

As a child, I learned that it wasn't okay to be angry. Back then, when that spiky little feeling started to scratch at the edges, I was supposed to simply hold my head up and "be positive," whatever that means. Smile and channel it into something productive, something appropriately aligned with the kinds of goals I was supposed to have. For me, that meant using my suppressed anger to fuel extreme athleticism which, as an adult, become a running addiction. I would smile and bite my tongue as I clocked mile after mile up hills and down, along windy shores and on city sidewalks and through winding forest trails.

Fitness is one thing, as is discipline and pushing through discomfort for the sake of a goal. But more often than not, I was pounding the ground beneath my feet day after day after day *instead of* dealing with whatever was bothering me. Instead of directly addressing a hurtful comment from my partner, I would say nothing and go put on my running shoes. Instead of saying no to an additional task at work, I'd agree then run until my knees ached. I didn't feel like I could set limits or that I had any control over the circumstances of my life, but I could always go for a run.

Then my back refused to allow me to move let alone exercise. I could no longer grit my teeth and sweat out my anger and, on top of that, I now had a truly maddening condition to manage. And so I got really, really mad, but without the usual outlet at my disposal. All those years' worth of things I hadn't said or done, or even admitted to myself, had been stacked one atop another, exerting more and more pressure, and now the only thing left to do was explode or collapse.

What I would later come to realize is that having anger about your circumstances is part of the healing process. It can be a fire under you that gets you out of bed, that makes you keep fighting. It can be a healthy part of your repair, your transformation. It can be the kind of heat that turns a million individual grains of sand into a cohesion of glass, that makes you speak your truth despite the consequences, that makes you stand up for yourself and others. Anger can be an extraordinary motivator against the great injustices of the world. Anyone who joined the Black Lives Matter movement after the acquittal of Trayvon Martin's killer, or anyone who walked in the Women's March on January 21, 2017, or anyone who was brought to tears by the video of environmental activist Greta Thunberg's speech at the UN can attest to that.

Yet anger with nowhere to go can become chronic, a chronic default setting that has the tendency to shift into victimhood. Consider the political outrage right now, people from all along the political spectrum manage to be the sole wronged party, the victims of the "evil" machinations of those on the other side of the aisle. *They are out to get me*, we think, then spend the next four hours spewing on the Internet. But who exactly is "they"?

As counterintuitive as it may seem, not only can identifying and behaving as a victim serve us, it can feel really, really good. If you have no personal power, then all you have to do is sit around, waiting for someone to swoop in and save you. In that way, it is a powerful role with tremendous benefits. As Dr. David Hanscom noted in his book, establishing yourself as a victim makes it so that others expect less of you, and you might even feel entitled to manipulate to get what you want because you are "right" and the world is wrong. Why bother trying to be good person when the world, your body, your life is out to get to you? Why bother trying at all?

Like so many people with a penchant for striving and chronic but unrecognized anger, I had never really found an appropriate outlet or a decent role model to talk to about the unattainability of and alternative to the American Dream. Now I couldn't stop thinking about the fact that I was a young woman in her athletic prime, unable to tie her own shoes or get even a moment's relief from all-consuming pain. It was so unfair.

But there is no "fair" when it comes to pain and, as I mentioned in the previous chapter, illness, injury, and trauma are not evenly distributed. This was new terrain for me. So used to being able to power through and deny, deny, deny what my body and my life were trying to tell me, I now found myself about as angry as I'd ever been. At a loss for how to manage my pain and limited mobility, and with my usual method of coping now unavailable, I was overwhelmed with a sense of victimhood. That is when I decided to simply opt out.

I am so incredibly lucky that my suicide attempt failed. I do not want to suggest that suicide is a necessarily stop on the path toward healing—it is decidedly *not*. Please do not do what I did. If you are thinking about taking action that can end your life, please reach out to for help. Call a friend, family member, colleague, your doctor or mental health therapist, or the National Suicide Prevention Lifeline (800-273-8255).

Clearly it wasn't my time to leave this world. Even so, when I woke up I was still mad. I still felt like a victim of circumstance. But my suicide attempt had killed a piece of my ego, and my inexplicable survival woke me up—I was ready to stop waiting and start doing something real about it.

FALLING APART AND TAKING RESPONSIBILITY

Falling apart in some form or another seems to be a common theme in stories of recovery. The phrase "hitting rock bottom" is used in Alcoholics Anonymous to describe people's very worst moments; the moments that were so horrific that it forced them to wake up. The terrible car accident they caused, or the family they broke up, or the violence they perpetrated or fell prey to—it was this and only this that got them to look at their lives and the role they played in it in a new way.

Obviously, this is not ideal. Wouldn't it be so much easier to stop and seek help before getting to the point of crisis? Of course it would. But we are creatures of routine, and if that routine is to go, go, go, or drink, drink, drink, then something extraordinary needs to happen to shake us loose.

Mine was attempted suicide, and the literal waking up was followed by the metaphorical waking up. Suddenly, I was ready to deal with my anger, my life, not as what I thought it should be but as what it actually was.

There could be any number of circumstances that brought you to read this book. Maybe you've been diagnosed with cancer, or hit by a car, or lived in an abusive relationship, or lost someone you loved more than anything in the world. Perhaps you have justifiable anger at the distracted physician, the drunk driver, the partner who used his fists to control. You might be mad at life or feel like a victim of life's cruelty. And that's okay.

Life has a brilliant way of bringing us all to our knees, both literally and figuratively. It is that moment when our knees hit the ground that our eyes open wide. It is here at the bottom, broken open, in the darkness of the unmapped territory of hopelessness, pain, fear, and anger, where a gateway to a new path might appear. As Brene Brown said, "Only when we are brave enough to explore the darkness will we discover the infinite power of our light."

ENDURING TRANSFORMATION

When I fight my pain, I am also fighting love; when I allow my pain, I can also allow love. And that allowing is transformative.

Not that transformation is ever a clean or easy process, direct or clear-cut. It is messy, rarely enjoyable (at least at the beginning), and often frustrating. It involves being brave enough to face your shadow, muddle through your own darkness and humanity's darkness while owning and integrating it without losing yourself.

If healing is about making contact with "all" of the self, of neither denying nor cutting off parts of who we are, then we must compassionately face our pain, wounding, and trauma. We must become a container of love and support. We must be willing to do the shadow work and find our way in the dark in order to reach the light, because the only way out is through. (Or as Robert Frost wrote, from the perspective of a exhausted farm wife with a never-ending list of chores to do in "A Servant to Servants," "I can see no way but through.")

Once we accept that, we become more fully connected to our own humanity and therefore, more fully connected with all of life. This is where true healing lies.

FINALLY, SURRENDER

When there's nowhere left to run, that which is determined to unfold will unfold. When there is no means to resist and nobody to blame, that is when we surrender.

I continually forget and remember the meaning of surrender. It is an elusive concept, an alchemy that can be more easily understood when compared with striving and dissatisfaction, victimhood and anger. It's easier to talk about what surrender is not: it is not weakness, failure, or defeat, not throwing in the towel or giving up. It is not succumbing to the negative internal narratives or darkness driven by fear. Nor is it pushing or straining or fighting against circumstance, not clenching or tightening, not flailing about for the next best strategy for escaping the present.

It lies somewhere in the middle. Or rather, it lies somewhere outside of this normal state of existence; in that place where we know that we can't continue to live as we have but we *don't know* what's next. Something has to change, but we're okay with not knowing the *how* and the *when*. It's a state of humility, a relaxing into the unknowability of existence, of letting go and turning inward. It's a motion as simple as the inhale and the exhale.

Some people call this state "flow." Some call it "God." Some call it unconditional love, or universal love, or simply "love." It is beyond desire, beyond attainment, beyond grasping or resisting; it is an acceptance of the finitude of the individual self and the infinitude of the self as part of the universe.

The art of surrender is learning how to flow, not clench.

There is an absolute trust that comes with surrendering to illness, injury, or trauma, when you allow your body/mind to go through what it needs to go through, trusting that whatever is unfolding is exactly what's supposed to happen. Once you truly surrender, an internal calmness amidst external chaos takes over, and a sense of unwavering trust begins to inhabit every part of your being. Trust in a higher reason, a higher intelligence to guide you. This higher intelligence is still you. It's the soul level part of the self, the spirit, the divine whisperer.

It is through that trust that you're able to get out of our own way, entering into a place of great spaciousness that gives rise to greater clarity and insight into co-creation with all of life, including your healing process. Life—you, your pain, the world—feels like a lazy river, of which you are a drop of water and the entire body of water, its motion and energy. Your job is to sit back, relax, and to let it take you wherever it goes, over the gentle shallows and the bumpy rapids with the same curiosity and acceptance.

Insight, creativity, and "Ah Ha" moments come through from this place. Here is where you can begin to access your intuition, your inner GPS that will guide the course of your healing process.

Reflection Questions

I'd like to invite you to take a deep breath and answer the following questions as honestly as possible.

- What societal expectations are important to you? Why?

- When have you sacrificed your health or personal values for the sake of others or to fulfill societal expectations?
- What do "healthy boundaries" mean to you? How capable are you of setting healthy boundaries? Where or when is it difficult for you to advocate for yourself?
- As a child, what were you taught about anger?
- When do you feel angry? What does anger feel like in your body?
- How do you manage anger? In what ways does your style of anger management serve you? In what ways does your style of anger management hurt you?
- When do you feel like a victim? What does that feel like in your body?
- What happens when you feel like a victim?
- What is your experience with surrender or "flow"?

CHAPTER 3

Syncing Your Internal GPS

"Trust your instincts to the end, though you can render no reason."

—*Ralph Waldo Emerson*

"There is no medical explanation as to why you are still alive," the doctor said. "But here you are."

Fuck, I thought. My plan had been so carefully crafted; I'd done my research and then some. *How in God's name am I not dead?*

I wasn't the only one who asked that question, and I wasn't the only one who couldn't come up with an answer. After a long stint in the ER, I was admitted to the psych ward. Over the next ten days I met more doctors, more nurses, and more psychologists who struggled to find a way to help. To make matters worse, I was assigned to a therapy group with chronically depressed people. *I am not depressed!* I thought, perhaps irrationally for someone who'd just attempted suicide. True, I felt completely blocked from any lightness, disconnected from the divine, trapped in an abyss with no way out in sight. At the same time, I truly believed that depression was not the issue—it wasn't that I didn't love life, exactly, it was that the pain made me forget that love. I didn't want to die; I just wanted some idea of what was happening with my body. I just wanted relief.

The cognitive behavioral therapy went in one ear and out the other because the pain required my full attention and left me with zero cognitive resources for anything else. The psychiatrist's theory was that I needed some tiny buffer against the agonizing pain before I could be safely released back into the wild. Finding a drug that actually worked so that I could get more than a couple consecutive hours of sleep would make a world of difference.

A day into my stay, I requested a visit from a hospital Buddhist chaplain. Something within me knew that I wasn't there just to find the right prescription, but that I needed some kind of spiritual medicine. These visits, more so than those with doctors and other medical specialists, would bring about healing.

"Katherine Hand, visitor in waiting room four," blared the hospital loudspeaker the next day. Perfect timing! This was my ticket out of therapy group, where a bunch of chronically depressed people were making each other more depressed. I limped down the hall, the pain just as bad as it had been before my suicide attempt, but I had a glimmer of hope in my heart.

I entered waiting room four and froze. There was the chaplain, but it was not just any chaplain. It was Tara, the kindest, most loving spiritual teacher I've ever known. We'd met years earlier at local meditation center, and she'd mentored me for a while when I was trying to integrate Buddhist meditation into my work. We hadn't seen each other for ages, but it felt like no time had passed. I looked into her eyes and she looked into mine our mouths hanging open, both utterly speechless. There was absolutely no one else on the planet with whom I would rather spend time in my traumatized state. She embodied compassion like that of a Buddha; holding space for deep love, care, and concern.

I knew in my bones that a higher intelligence had coordinated our meeting. In her presence I could let go of my obsession with diagnoses and problem solving; mostly we sat together in silence. Other times Tara asked me questions. What was my relationship with pain? How was I treating myself; with love and compassion or with anger and force? We talked some, about my identification with being able-bodied. What would happen if I couldn't define myself in the ways I had before?

Before her arrival, I'd felt like I'd been forsaken by God, but now I was back in the flow of life, reconnected with the divine. Even when facing the hardest of questions, I felt like a child being held by her mother; surrounded by softness and love. Knowing she was in my life, I was ready to move forward, come what may.

Not that I'd let go of my desire to figure out what was going on once I was released from the psych ward, with a new medication that miraculously allowed me to sleep for a few hours at a time. As much as I could practice surrendering to my new circumstances, I still wanted an explanation and a detailed road map. (This is part of the continual forgetting and remembering process—there are moments when you can remember to be OK with not being OK, and there are moments when you just can't.) I was still anxious, obsessive even, about healing my body and relieving my pain.

As winter turned to spring, I saw a melange of, doctors, nurses, and alternative health practitioners with little luck. Many of these professionals seemed narrow-sighted and full of ego, more interested in a set of symptoms than me as a whole person with a complicated life. Fortunately for me, Karen, an amazing physical therapist, had made it her personal mission to conquer my complex case. She insisted that I look for new doctors and referred me to someone whom I would come to view as an angel in a white lab coat.

My new doctor, Dr. Macadam, was otherworldly, like an ancient Shaman healer who happened to have been reincarnated as a traditional medical doctor. To her my pain wasn't a stand-alone symptom, it was part of a system in which every part was connected. She just got it.

After several visits we began to figure things out. During one of our initial meetings, she walked in and handed me Dr. David Hanscom's book *Control: A Spine Surgeons Roadmap Out of Chronic Pain.* "Take a look at this," she said.

No fucking way, echoed throughout my mind. This was the same book my boss had given me to read just before I got injured. It was in that moment that I knew I was exactly where I was supposed to be. That thought allowed surrender, which paradoxically allowed me to take the lead in my recovery process.

In hindsight, it was clear the universe had been giving me whispers and signals months prior to my injury, preparing me for what lie ahead. Beginning with my blossoming friendship with Amanda, who served as an example of how to move through life with grace after having sustained massive physical trauma, to the arrival of Tara in the psych ward, to this book by David Hanscom that kept reappearing. On the flip side, I'd been unconsciously relaying whispers and signals to the universe through my thoughts and intentions. From seeing the man moving from his wheelchair to his vehicle outside my new apartment building and thinking over and over how I could never go on without the ability to move independently, to begging the universe for circumstances that would allow me to quit my research job so I could write books and give inspirational talks. How could these coincidences and serendipities not be divinely orchestrated by a higher intelligence?

The greatest lesson from all of this was of learning to be more synchronized with all of life. We are not separate particles operating in the world independently from one another, but rather within a higher orchestration beyond our awareness or understanding. A cough in Chile and a fight in Norway and a hug in China will reach us eventually.

Once we can surrender to this divine intelligence, we can begin to see that everything works for our good, even in the midst of great chaos, pain, trauma, injury or illness. We can remain open and available to the divine whispers echoing around and within us, and to look deeply and with clear discernment. To find that the most powerful healer lies within.

LOOKING WITHOUT

Before there were doctors in white lab coats, there were shamans and medicine men, priests and midwives and herbalists. Just like today, some of these people were patient and thoughtful, taking the time to listen and look at each individual as their own unique universe. Some were superstitious following rules without making an effort to understand them or ask themselves whether they were worth following. Some were aggressive and full of ego and used medicine to prove and promote themselves to the detriment of those they were meant to help. Some were simply snake oil salespeople looking to turn a profit, buyer be damned.

There were also all kinds of patients. Some wanted an easy answer from a figure of authority. Some were willing to work for healing through a long-term care relationship. Some paused and looked within.

For most of my life, I was the first kind of patient. If you had a white lab coat and a stethoscope looped around your neck, I would have eaten my own socks if you told me it would make me feel better. After all, I knew nothing, and doctors knew everything.

Many of us have been taught that someone in a white lab coat knows more about our bodies after spending twenty minutes with us than we do. Sometimes that can be blessedly true, like when a doctor can pop a dislocated shoulder back in place or identify your mystery rash as pityriasis (not measles) at a glance and prescribe rest, lots of fluids, an oatmeal bath, and a topical corticosteroid if necessary. We certainly have many good reasons to venerate modern medicine—the scientific method, though fallible, has led to some groundbreaking discoveries. Penicillin, the polio vaccine, and Cesarean sections have saved countless lives, as have X-Rays, MRIs, and defibrillators. Even handwashing—imagine where we would be without Dr. Ignaz Semmelweis's thorough investigation of hospital-acquired infection and intervention.[2] However, the trouble begins when we give away all personal power to what has become an incredibly complex, sometimes impersonal, often for-profit industry. There are many good reasons not to trust doctors just as there are many good reasons not to trust *people*. Doctors-as-people and the medical establishment-at-large can have ulterior motives, biases, and blind spots, just like everyone else.

It is impossible for anyone to know everything, and sometimes the best-intentioned medical professionals overlook evidence and make egregious, even life-threatening, mistakes. That being said, there is also ample evidence of discrimination, ignorance, greed, and downright cruelty in medicine. The Tuskegee experiment, in which so-called researchers from the U.S. Public Health Service didn't treat 500 black sharecroppers for syphilis even after the discovery of a cure,[3] is perhaps the most well-known example. They claimed to be studying the progression of the disease, even though its terrible outcome was already well documented.

That was cruelty in action. Then there's oversight through ignorance and discrimination: real studies, ones that are sincerely meant to better understand conditions and their treatment, often seem to forget about the existence of women. Cardiovascular disease is the number one killer of women, yet less than a third of clinical trials include female patients.[4]

Currently big in the news is the systemic dismissal of women's pain and other symptoms, or "health-care gaslighting"—even Serena Williams, one of the most famous athletes in the world and a woman of color, nearly died from a pulmonary embolism after giving birth because the nurse discounted her distress.[5] Today black infants are more than twice as likely to die than white infants,[6] a long-standing racial disparity attributed to a disparity in care.

Even when racism and sexism aren't a factor, money can be. Look to the opioid crisis, which was declared a public health emergency in 2017 after causing hundreds of thousands of deaths[7] and untold economic and community damage, as the profits of pharmaceutical companies profits. No wonder people are wary of the medical establishment!

I can't tell you when to trust experts and when not to. That's what makes this topic so tricky—it is so, so difficult to know. I've certainly fallen prey to unscrupulous practitioners. Remember the alternative medical practitioner who treated me for four years after I fell down the stairs in 2012? She told me that she was the *only* person who could help me, and that if I quit seeing her and paying her $250-per-session fee, the concussion would return. Then, when I got hurt in 2016, she saw me for two sessions after which she told me over the phone that she couldn't see me anymore. I'd started stepping out on her by seeing a neurologist for the pain. When she found out, she dropped me as her patient.

Since then I've wondered if she was worried that he would see some red flags about her treatment, including her possessiveness.

My back injury would eventually teach me that as a general rule, doctors don't always know best. Some do, some don't. Some are open, curious, and knowledgeable; some are cynical and narrow-minded and overextended. This applies to healers of other modalities. I lucked out by meeting Tara, an extraordinary Buddhist chaplain, who helped me by pushing me to question my beliefs and providing a loving space in which I could be quiet and listen. Of course not all chaplains, Buddhist or otherwise, would have had such a profound impact on me.

The only two adages that can generally apply to getting solid help are "It depends" and "Educate yourself." The onus falls on you to heal yourself by reading the latest research from reputable sources, thoroughly vetting the medical professionals in your life, and making the time to practice tapping in to your internal GPS. The question is, how do you tap in?

INTUITION: YOUR INTERNAL GPS

As you travel down the path of healing, you will need to partner with those who have worked hard to become professionals in the field of healing and medicine. These people will have information that may be key to your healing process but, at the same time, you are the top primary physician of your own well-being. While modern medicine is an absolute blessing and an essential tool at your disposal, don't forget your own healing intuition. Blending the two will enable you to further your healing process.

Scientific research has shown the benefits of using intuition with conventional medical knowledge. Dr. Kelley Turner spent years traveling across the world talking with cancer survivors, people who had healed against all odds. Through her research she identified nine key factors present in those who survived the advanced stages of cancer. One of these key factors was their ability to use their intuition to help make decisions related to their healing process. (Kelly A. Turner, 2014)

Even without a life-threatening illness, you can benefit from the messages within you. Remember, only you live inside your body. Your consciousness, that thing that makes you you, includes the sensations of your body, inside and out, gross and subtle, tangible and intangible. Even the space inside your body that feels dark or inaccessible is actually filled with conscious awareness and you can, to some degree, detect the same space as a medical instrument, MRI, or bloodwork. For example, a year after my injury I literally didn't know how to move my body. I couldn't get from point A to point Z without injuring myself. The long duration of acute pain had basically rewired my motor cortex. The doctor sent me to Feldenkrais movement therapy, where I began to learn how to sense different parts of my body. Over time my mind/body connection became more and more refined, and I could sense the subtleties going on in my body and begin to rewire my brain so I could walk again. One side effect of this therapy was that my body awareness became heightened to the point that when I came down with a sinus infection, I could tell the doctor exactly what was going on (right sphenoid sinus blocked) without needing an MRI.

This is possible because you and your body are one. Mind and body are one. Anxiety, for example, is the physical experience of shaking hands or a tight chest, the emotional and cognitive experience of fear or worry, and even an experience within the realm of philosophy, an existential dread. Where is the line between these experiences? There is none. This concept lies at the very foundation of holistic medicine.

A direct feedback loop between mind and body exists within you. Even using such a description doesn't quite cut it because it implies separation. The point is that the feedback loop ties to a beautiful navigating system that, when we allow it, serves to guide us along our path. Many call this "intuition," a word whose definition is nebulous and yet felt by many. I believe that intuition is our organic divinity that keeps us safe from harm and in alignment with our higher purpose. It's the small voice inside leading us towards truth and healing. There are various levels of intuition within us:

GUT INSTINCT

The first is gut instinct, which operates as an immediate reaction to perceived eminent danger. In scientific terms, this would be categorized as the sympathetic nervous system (part of the autonomous nervous system), which is responsible for the elevated breathing rate, the flush of blood to the extremities, and a shot of oxygen to the brain in the flight-or-fight response. This is simple survival intuition, a primitive operating system that is always on whether we're aware of it or not.

A glitch in gut instinct is that it can become overly sensitive or inappropriately activated. A single car accident can make every car ride thereafter an exercise in controlled panic. Getting mugged once can lead to cringing every time a stranger approaches on the street. The definitively non-fatal prospect of public speaking can increase heart rate just like proximity to the edge of a cliff.

Which means gut instinct is neither good nor bad. Sometimes it saves us, sometimes it causes undo stress.

INNER GUIDANCE

Inner guidance is neither gut instinct or intellectual discernment, though there may be elements of one or both. It is neither animal response or the stilted response of conditioning. So what exactly is it?

That is a tremendously difficult question to answer, in no large part because it is a phenomenon of experience, and that experience is different for everyone. For some it is a feeling in the back of the neck or in the belly, or the sensation of energy moving from the heart to the hands. For some it is a singular voice inside the head. For some it is the relationship to the sun or moon or rain. (See the next section for more on intuition and how to cultivate it.)

Whatever the experience, intuition is about integrity and self-respect; a unity between listening, discerning, and acting on the divine information that manifests within you. It is a trust that your inner voice is here to serve your highest good, even when there's no obvious logic to the guidance you're receiving.

OBSTACLES TO ACCESSING INTUITION

Where does insecurity, need for approval, and fear come from? For most of us, the internalized voices of disapproval, often speaking so softly they are below our conscious awareness, come from lived experiences. It could be the voice of a disciplinarian father, or a judgmental mother, or an overburdened teacher, a commercial on TV. All those magazines you read as a teenager, magazines that taught you that your hair was wrong, your body was wrong, and that no boy would like you until you made them right—those magazines can continue to hold jurisdiction over your sense of self if not actively managed.

Then there are the voices of the loving father, the gentle mother, the kind teacher, the profound book that taught you the nuances of morality, the value of sharing, and how pro-social behavior is both good and personally beneficial. Those voices are essential to your successfully navigating the world in an ethical, efficient way.

Egoic authority is neither bad nor good. Developing awareness and attunement to these voices, as well as intellectual discernment so they aren't running the show or gripping your attention, will give you freedom of choice, freedom from the ego's reign. You get to decide what to listen to and what to dismiss.

INTUITION AND TRAUMA

Trauma is any deeply distressing experience that has occurred in the past and which, if unrecognized and unmanaged, can have an ongoing and profound impact on the present. There is no such thing as a trauma free life. Everyone experiences trauma meaning it's common and, it's ideally, an opportunity for growth and shared healing. If you don't have enough trauma in your life, you can look to your ancestors—the jury is out on whether trauma is passed down through the generations via altered gene expression versus altered behavior but, either way, your parents' hurt and their parents' hurt and their parents' hurt will reach you somehow. Hopefully the continued study of epigenetics will bring us closer to answers around nature versus nurture and, of course, what we can do about it.

Trauma can leave an imprint of itself on the body/mind. To use a computer analogy, trauma can cause a rewriting of the nervous system's code. I say *can* because it totally depends on the individual person. An event that could completely shake me up might be no big deal to you.

Because trauma can impact you on a level below consciousness, managing it is not always a cognitive process. It can certainly be helpful to think through an event (especially compared to trying to avoid or deny it), and many find the support of a trained therapist to be beneficial. Cognitive Processing Therapy (CPT) and Prolonged Exposure Therapy (PET) both involve, cognitive processing. Other therapies, like Eye Movement Desensitization and Reprocessing (EMDR) and Stress Inoculation Training (SIT) are less about examining the event or events and more about developing methods to modulate feelings around it. All of these therapies can be incredibly helpful for different people at different times.

In moments of dysregulation related to trauma, reaching out to someone, whether a professional or a friend or partner, to help you regulate your nervous system can be invaluable. This is what Tara did for me. She facilitated my calming so that I could face myself, my pain, and my situation head on. In this way, the Internal GPS isn't only a "me" system but a "we" system; her mere presence allowed me to sync up with a calmer, clearer state of being. Just like there's no distinct line between body and mind, there is no distinct line between within and without. Together we can find the collective current of life.

Emotional regulation and bringing awareness into the body can be part of the practice of developing intuition. When we allow ourselves to feel into the body, we plug into the most physical aspect of our Internal GPS. We ground ourselves, drop into the senses, and listen. This activates our intuition and makes space for healing and innovation.

Intuition Check: *A quick and easy way to recognize intuition is by checking whether or not your current mind/ body experience can be described by the following adjectives.*

- **Intuition is NOT:** fearful, panicked, critical, judgmental, blaming, punishing, angry, emotionally charged.
- **Intuition is:** neutral, detached, calm, objective, peaceful and subtle.

AWAKENING INTUITION

I for one tend to think my way through life. I like to weigh the pros and cons before coming to a decision, which serves me well when those pros and cons can be clearly defined. But what about those times when there are too many unknowns to apply logic?

If our brains are the only muscle we're exercising, then we're going to struggle when it can't come to a solution. The danger of moving through the world in a cognition-centric, disembodied way is that we allow our divine guidance system to atrophy, and so it is weak or out of practice when we really need it.

Awakening your healing intuition is a matter of recovering a skill that already lies within. Like information readily accessible over the internet, your healing intuition is always available. You just need the correct IP address to tap it. Holistic healers can help you harness and unblock subtle energies, often referred to as qi or prana, that can help lead you there. Ultimately it's up to you to find it.

Like any skill, it's never too late to start developing intuition. All it takes is practice, practice, practice!

First, we must inhabit an embodied sense of self. Like most things health and healing related, we can't use force, worry, or attachment to an outcome to "make it happen." Rather, you want to create the conditions in your internal and external environment that allow you to hear the subtle whispers of your intuitive voice. From this place, we can begin to recognize what intuition is, and what it is not. Since intuition is often very subtle, it's easiest to recognize when the mind is calm and quiet.

In a fast-paced world where we're constantly stimulated, I've found practices such a yoga, qi gong, tai chi, prayer, journaling, quiet contemplation, energy healing, meditation, tapping points, reiki, hypnosis, biofeedback, Ayurvedic message, ecstatic dance, and time in nature helpful. Each of these methods are meant to facilitate a sense of spaciousness and connection with the body. I recommend engaging in at least one of your chosen methods every day. Spend a few minutes devoted to listening to this voice. The emerging wisdom may appear as a hunch, an image, a gut feeling, a sound, a memory, or an instant knowing as if a light bulb was suddenly switched on. Learn to trust the signals your inner wisdom sends, then most importantly, act on them!

In the following sections, I will discuss how to use body/mind practices, dreams, mediation, and journaling to awaken the connection to your divine inner wisdom.

TAI CHI AND OTHER BODY/MIND AWARENESS PRACTICES

Tai Chi allowed me to heal what modern medicine couldn't. In all honesty, I didn't really want to take tai chi, because I didn't understand what the two-thousand-year-old healing practice entailed and frankly, at the time it seemed to me like a lot of hocus pocus. But the divine whispers were loud and clear, so I hesitantly enrolled myself in a series of 8 a.m. classes.

I soon discovered that tai chi is all about awareness and intuition. During the class the teacher gently pointed out problematic patterns of movement and adjusted my posture and style of shifting the body. She told me that it was okay to lean into the painful parts of my body and showed me how to do so without clenching or guarding. Under her careful direction, I began to feel my body relax and I got a sense of how normal movement felt.

I'd tried just about every modern medical treatment for my condition over the course of three years, yet it took only one class for me to feel different. With Tai Chi I could feel the inside space of my body and draw upon my own innate ability to heal myself.

Tai Chi worked well for me, but it's only one of many modalities that work to build physical and mental awareness and strength. Yoga, qi gong, and martial arts fall into this category, as does any form of movement—that is, if the practitioner's intention is not aggressive pushing or superficial body image goals but rather focus and listening.

MEDITATION

Many people have their strongest intuitive insights during meditation. One of my best friends attended a ten-day silent meditation retreat, at the end of which her intuitive voice said, "Start a healing dance community." As soon as she got home, she quit her job and turned a new page, devoting her life to creating a community that has been thriving for twenty years.

Attending a lengthy meditation retreat is not necessary to begin accessing your intuitive voice. You can begin with a guided meditation CD, joining a local mediation group, or start practicing independently. You can go on a walk in the woods, with no cell phone or other distraction and with the intention to focus on the natural world around you. Really, you can set the timer on your phone for 3 minutes and just sit still—that's meditation.

You can also create some structure by giving yourself a point of focus for your meditation. You can repeat a prayer or phrase (mantra), such as "I am love" or "May all beings be happy and free." You can ask a question of the universe, feeling it deeply in your heart. You might get an answer such as *yes* or *not now* or *I love you so much, I'm not going to give you this.* You might get silence, at least for the time being. Practice welcoming any answer or non-answer with compassion and calm.

JOURNALING

Oftentimes people successfully access the intuitive parts of their brain using carefully selected journal questions. Once you've decided on a question, begin writing and don't stop. Don't think about or analyze the question in your rational mind; simply let the word river flow through your fingertips. If you develop writer's block, write about the block until it's cleared. Just don't stop writing. The goal is to bypass the logical mind and get into a "flow "state of consciousness, thereby developing direct access to intuition and divine insights within you.

Reflection Questions

I'd like to invite you to take a deep breath and answer the following questions as honestly as possible.

- Where in the body does my intuition live?
- Is my intuitive voice soft and subtle or loud and vigorous?
- What blocks me from following my intuition?
- Is my need for control getting in the way of listening to my intuition?

- Where is my intuition guiding me on my healing journey?
- Is it guiding me towards or away from specific healers?
- Am I willing to let go of knowing how my journey will unfold in order to follow the trail of bread-crumbs guided by intuition?

CHAPTER 4

Finding Faith

"The power that made the body, heals the body."—B. J. Palmer

For two years after my suicide attempt, I tirelessly pursued healing. I went to appointment after appointment, making a little progress here and there, regressing there and here. In other words, two uneven, painful steps forward, one uneven, painful step back. I did my long list of physical therapy exercises every morning, took my anti-inflammatories religiously, did my best not to complain and to exude an outward sunniness, no matter how I really felt inside. Tara, the Buddhist chaplain, had given me a sense of loving acceptance, but it's hard to hold on to that feeling when pain is shrieking like a fire alarm. Every now and then I'd remember to sit quietly and allow my heart to soften, but mostly I reverted to my default setting of taking action and working hard. Overall, progress was happening, but it was slow like molasses, painfully, soul-crushingly slow.

One morning I limped into First Hill Swedish Medical Center, right off Columbia Street and Boren Avenue, in the neighborhood known locally as "pill hill" because of its high concentration of hospitals. My doctor's appointment went as doctor's appointments usually did; an assessment of the pain, a recommendation to keep doing what I was already doing, a future time set to check in yet again. Not much got done, and the doctor seemed as wearied by the process as I was. These appointments tended to leave me depressed, and that day was no different.

Afterward, I walked out onto the sidewalk along Boren Avenue, a busy thoroughfare that runs from the International District to South Lake Union and bisects Capitol Hill from downtown. I don't recall if the day was sunny or rainy, just that my internal weather was bleak. Then I looked up. A couple blocks to the west two towers reached their gray-green domes into the sky. Something told me that I should head in that direction.

The cathedral was grand and ancient, at least in comparison to the other buildings in this relatively new city. Above the big bronze doors, a black-and-gold window depicted Jesus with his arms spread wide and the words, "I am the vine, you are the branches."

I am not a Catholic, but rather than being intimidated by the stately architecture and religious imagery, I felt a pull; a welcoming. I walked up the stairs and opened the bronze door. A glimpse inside took my breath away. A font stood in the expansive entryway and behind it, there were rows of polished wooden pews lined up in front of a white marble altar set in black slate. Stain-glass windows and simple globe chandeliers created a soft golden light; a high domed ceiling of gold plate and white spanned the space.

There is a reason why people used to spend so many resources on religious centers. The awesomeness—in the original sense of the word—simply inspires just as it is meant to do. Being in St. James Cathedral gave me a sense of the divine, what I and many others call God for lack of a way to describe the indescribable.

I took off my shoes and in my socks, padded down the center aisle. Off to the side was a little nook with a statue of Mary holding baby Jesus who in turn was holding an apple in his little hand. Rows of beeswax candles along the three walls lit the space and filled it with a sweet honey scent. Above, gold stars were painted onto the ceiling.

A dark-haired woman was kneeling in front of Mary, weeping and clutching a rosary in her hand. She looked up as I entered, and I placed my hand over my heart, then knelt down beside her and closed my eyes.

God, I prayed silently, *I am going to continue to do what I have to do every day, but I've been doing it for so long and it's so slow. I'm doing the work, but I need guidance. I don't know what else to do. I need your help.* A sense of movement, of giving myself over to something bigger than myself, of gratitude and peace, filled me. *Please*, I prayed. *I am open, I am open, I am open.*

After what could have been a minute or an hour, a priest walked by. I got up and followed him out of the church and into the courtyard. Usually, I wouldn't just run up to any old priest, especially since I am not a Catholic. But there was something about him, a humility and a kindness, that drew me toward him. "Father?" I said. "My name is Kat. Your church is so beautiful. I . . . I am not a Catholic, but . . . well, gosh. It's just so beautiful."

He nodded and smiled. "Welcome Kat. I'm Father Ryan." Emboldened, I continued, "Father Ryan, thank you. I hurt myself a couple years ago, and I've been in excruciating pain ever since. Nothing seems to really help all that much, or not for long. I'm wondering, do you do hands-on healing?"

"Yes Kat I do. If you call my secretary, he will help you schedule a session."

I went in for a session two weeks later, and I continued to go to the church on and off for about a year. It wasn't just the beauty of the place or the kindness and care of Father Ryan and the other priests and nuns who worked there—it was the inclusiveness, something I was not expecting from a Catholic Church or really, any religious institution. Across the street, St. James ran a homeless shelter that served three meals a day and offered mental health counseling, housing assistance, and clothing drives. On any given day, I might see a homeless person who'd come inside the sanctuary to get out of the rain near one of Seattle's wealthiest people sitting alone in a pew. Everyone was welcome, including me.

Every time I went into St. James Cathedral, I prayed, asking for help and surrendering myself to this unnamable power. Though I loved theory and structure and a clear-cut strategy, I was able to set all that aside and give myself over to the mystical, allowing it to unfold within me. As that God energy, that Jesus or Mary or whomever consciousness filled me, I felt my body drop into alignment. In those moments, my pain would cease.

Not long after I made the life-changing decision to walk into that church, I went out to lunch with a friend. Over savory pho and hot tea, she told me that she'd organized a seven-day silent meditation retreat at a bed and breakfast in the heart of Capitol Hill. The spiritual teacher would be flying out from Germany the day after tomorrow. Did I want to come?

At that time, sitting was a big challenge and was a position I could hold for only short periods, and even that usually caused a flare up. Still I registered and a couple days later, I was knocking on the door of a B&B down the street from Volunteer Park.

Some spiritual teachers can be pretty out of touch. All those hours spent alone in meditation and prayer is not conducive to keeping up with the zeitgeist. But this teacher, Marcus, was similar to Father Ryan, in that he had a humble, welcoming presence. He seemed genuinely interested in us. After dinner on the first night, he stood up and said, "We are going to be silent for the next six days." Those were the last words spoken.

For the next week, we woke up early, sat for an hour, did a walking mediation, had a "free" meditation in which we chose the style and venue, and then repeated that pattern throughout the day. We sat for a total of seven hours daily, an incredible feat for someone with a pain-free body, let alone me. The thing is, the more I sat, the more relaxed I became, and the more relaxed I became, the more my pain dissipated, and dissipated, and dissipated. During the walking meditations, I discovered that my limp, which I'd dragged with me for two years straight, had somehow disappeared, and my gaze focused forward, rather than on the ground at my feet. I felt so good that I forgot to take my anti-inflammatory medications and even forgot to drink water.

On the fourth day, a crisp, sunny February afternoon, I took myself on a walk up to Volunteer Park during free meditation. The leaves on the trees were greener, the sky bluer, the cherry blossom buds pinker. I swear, the birds were chirpier than they ever had been before. Suddenly, I heard someone call my name. I turned around and saw a fit blonde woman, a physical therapist at Swedish Medical Center who had worked with me immediately after my injury.

"Is that you Kat?" she said, a stunned expression on her face. A tear ran down her cheek.

I smiled and cleared the cobwebs from my throat. "Yes, I'm in the middle of a silent retreat," I said.

She nodded, wiped the tear away, and patted my shoulder. "You're moving . . . perfectly," she said.

THE POWER OF FAITH

Have you ever played with one of those giant multicolored playground parachutes? You know, the kind where one person lies down in the middle of the parachute, and everyone else forms a circle and holds the edge of the cloth. Then they lift the cloth together so that the person is suspended in it like a big hammock. On the count of three, everyone hoists the parachute so that the person goes flying up in the air, only to land in the center again, safely cradled. It is so much fun to be that person flying and falling, flying and falling.

I think of surrender and faith like being in the center of a playground parachute. When you fall back, confident that you will be caught—that is surrender. When you fly up in an explosion of energy—that is faith. It is like an assumption, without a specific direction or goal.

In that metaphor, faith is aligned with positive feelings: the joy of flight and expansiveness. We have faith that things *will* work out somehow. We might not have any idea of the exact route this working out will take, but we have faith in it anyway. We have faith in the power of miracles, the power of infinite possibilities. We have faith that we are being taken care of, that we will heal and love and be safe in the embrace of the divine.

It is not always that way. People often proclaim that they don't have faith, but there's no such thing as a faithless person. Faith is an expression of consciousness. The problem is that we misapply our faith. We tend to have more faith in the power of disaster than in the power of possibility. We all have faith of some kind, but for many of us, we have faith that things *will not* work out. Below our cognitive awareness might lie an assumption that we are alone in a dark cold universe, that we are weak and disease is strong, or that life is hard and we are as soft and vulnerable like a sleeping kitten. We have faith in the inevitability of relationships failing or that a decent income will always be out of reach. We have more faith in a disease's ability to kill us than we have in the power of a divine healing force.

There is good reason to be more attuned to negative information, what is sometimes referred to as the negativity bias. It comes down to survival. A study at Yale found that babies as young as three months paid more attention to negative social information that to positive social information,[8] which makes sense—as just about the most helpless creatures on earth, far more helpless than the newborns of almost every other species, it is critical for babies to pay attention to the moods of their caretakers. (What exactly they can do with that information at three months old isn't clear, beyond practicing for a future time when they will have more agency.) Young and working adults seem to be less motivated by positive framing than negative framing when assigned tasks,[9] despite what proponents of positive reinforcement might say. Really, all you have to do is read a newspaper or turn on the news—disaster, tragedy, and misbehavior draw a much wider audience than stories of people doing their best and getting along. There is something within us that gravitates toward disaster, be it right around the bend or all the way across the globe. That's because our very survival depends on seeing danger, whether it's in the form of a parent's oncoming rage, an oncoming truck, or an oncoming economic recession. (Fortunately, studies also show that the negativity bias can decrease with mindfulness practice[10] and age.[11] Perhaps once you've survived enough rages, trucks, and recessions, you no longer need to be so focused on danger.)

Assuming the knife can cut you when you're chopping a big juicy tomato or assuming that driving on an icy road can lead to a car accident is just plain smart. The problem arises, however, when danger is all we see, or when we assume danger well in advance of any signs of it, or we cling to negative narratives from the past rather than being open to a more positive future. Faith in the negative is myopic; it sees only a particular set of options. Faith turned toward the positive can be visionary; it sees infinite possibilities.

YOU HAVE TO ASK, IT'S THAT SIMPLE

Faith has a huge impact on your ability to heal and recover from disease, injury, or trauma, and so it is incredibly important how you choose to invest your faith. When you get a diagnosis, do you automatically assume the worst-case scenario is the correct one? Or do you assume that, no matter how dismal the odds, you will be one of that 10 percent of people who recovers?

Just as it's a whole lot easier to lie down on the couch when we're feeling tired, it's easier to get bad news and slip into a downward spiral. But faith, like most things, requires practice, and we must hone our attitudinal muscles through spiritual exercise, just like we hone our physical muscles through push-ups and squats.

The universe provides endless opportunities to practice, to choose aloneness versus connection, despair versus hope, victimhood versus responsibility. In the present moment we always have the opportunity to declare that the past is the past. This is now and through the grace of God/the divine/spirit/ whatever you want to call it, we are moving forward. Onward and upward!

I don't have a name for that something in which we put our faith. Anyway, names don't matter; all the world's religious texts and spiritual teachers are talking about the same thing. You could also argue, for that matter, that psychologists and economists and political scientists and every other "ist" has a different word for *it* too, whatever *it* is that somehow manages to organize chaos. But I digress. The point is this, in that moment kneeling before Mary in St. James Cathedral, I knew with ultimate certainty that there was a higher power beyond what my mind could fathom. *Something* had kept me alive. *Something* had returned Buddhist chaplain Tara to my life. *Something* was pushing me to continue with my healing work, through every setback and mistake and moment of agonizing pain. *Something* had carried me into that church.

Suddenly, faith dawned within me. Suddenly, I didn't feel so alone. I'd never thought too hard about it before—I worked hard, ran hard, checked off all the boxes on my adulting to-do list. Now that I was given the unwanted gift of having to stop doing things the way I had always done them, I could catch these moments of wonder more and more frequently. What was this *something* anyway?

Now that this unnamed something was with me and beyond me, I recognized a particular sticking point: I had been trying to heal myself all on my own. I'd been carrying the entire burden of not just this injury but my life on my back, which had both literally and figuratively fallen apart. I had always been the helper, the one who would drop everything to support a partner, colleague, or friend. That's not a bad thing, in moderation and, more importantly, with reciprocation. The problem was that I didn't know how to ask for help, how to be the "helpee" when I needed support. Now that this injury had forced me to need support and need it desperately, I was getting a lot of practice asking for help. Doctors, physical therapists, Buddhist chaplains, psychiatrists, energy healers, and an orthopedic dentist had all come to my aid when I let them. My intuition came to my aid, too—when I'd asked myself for guidance. But there was one source of help, that I hadn't yet tapped.

As a product of our modern Western culture that lauds independence above all else, I had never considered the idea to "simply ask" a higher power for assistance. Honestly, it hadn't even occurred to me. But many of my friends and spiritual teachers began pointing me in a certain direction: the direction of prayer. Meanwhile, beautiful stories about people who had experienced miraculous healings by simply asking the divine for help began to flood into my life. *There must be something too this,* I thought, happy to be actually paying attention and listening to the divine whispers as they arrived.

We're so conditioned to looking frantically for solutions, to trying to make things happen, that asking for help doesn't even occur to us. The point is that we must stop taking on the entire burden of our healing process and simply ask for help, with the faith that our prayers will be heard and answered. It doesn't matter "who" your prayers are sent to; just send them out with a sincere heart and wait patiently for them to be answered while continuing to take responsibility for your healing process. The more you can stay centered within the transformational energies of life, the more your life will transform, with you taking initiative to seize opportunity when it comes.

I was certainly allowing for the mystery of miracles to unfold in my life, while simultaneously taking ownership and responsibility for my recovery process. The next step was to ask for help and have faith, beyond a shadow of a doubt, that the higher intelligence guiding all of life would help my body to heal. The week at that silent meditation retreat was the next phase of letting go, of clearing the way for divinity to find me. Which it did.

I would go on to meet a spiritual teacher who would give me a prayer that proved powerful in my healing process. "Go home and enter into silent prayer tonight," she would tell me. "Say to the divine: 'I'm no longer safe in my body. My body is no longer my home, it's your home. I have done everything I know to make it good again. Please keep my home safe and help it to become healthy again.' Then, let go."

For several weeks after meeting her, my recovery stayed the same, but every night I prayed before I went to bed. I would lie down and enter into silent meditative prayer and, once my mind was quiet, I would feel a deep sense of peace and tranquility, a sensation of gentle warmth flowing through my body. From the depth of my heart, I asked the divine for help in the way the spiritual teacher had described.

Then, slowly but surely, everything began to change.

FINDING FAITH

I am one of those people who is very comfortable with investigating and incorporating a variety of healing modalities and religious or spiritual practices. In my experience, no practices is *the* true practice. Every practice has the potential to be true to someone. Plenty of people who hold firm to a particular belief system might disagree, and I welcome that disagreement. All I can do is describe what has been meaningful to me.

That being said, there are beautiful prayers from different spiritual practices around the world. Jewish prayers, Muslim prayers, Buddhist prayers, Hindu prayers, Catholic and Sufi prayers . . . the list goes on and on. Everywhere, it seems, people have codified praise of and requests from their particular god or gods, have chanted and sang and whispered the same prayers over and over again for thousands of years. (In a perfect world, this human impulse would bring us together rather than tear us apart.) You can take any or all of them; leave any or all of them. You might also find that it makes much more sense to talk casually to whomever or whatever it is you want to talk to, to have a casual conversation with mystery, to send a message from the heart—that works too.

Reflection Questions

I'd like to invite you to take a deep breath and answer the following questions as honestly as possible.

- Do you tend to be more pessimistic or more optimistic? Do you tend to have faith in disaster, or faith in infinite possibility?
- What is your experience with faith and prayer?
- What is your relationship with God/the divine? What word do you use for the mystical?
- How do you feel about asking the divine for help?
- If you were to ask for help from the mystical, what would you say?

CHAPTER 5

The Momentum of Belief

"Whatever the mind can conceive it can achieve."—W. Clement Stone

In all honesty, I didn't expect anything dramatic to happen. After what felt like an eternity living with pain, I'd come to think of myself as a sick, frail person. Every time I stepped outside, I was paranoid that people would see me limping and judge me as a sick, frail person. (Of course, that was just a projection. I'm sure that people walking down the street had more important things on their minds than my limp!) Because I identified as a sick, frail person, I made the choices of a sick, frail person, walking only on familiar terrain and, besides my many doctors' appointments, sticking mostly close to home. Managing pain was my life, and I was afraid of anything and everything that posed even the slightest threat to aggravate it. My world had become smaller and smaller, as had my self-concept.

Each of the traditional medical professionals I'd been working with indicated that it would take at least ten years to regain somewhat normal functioning, at best. I understood the concept of neuroplasticity from my research background, and so I knew that rewiring the brain is an elusive process that takes time. So many of the patients in that study of chronic pain on which I'd been working before my own injury had lost patience, a response I could relate to all too well.

I'd begun to cultivate faith in a healing force that would support my recovery through prayer and meditation, and often I believed in my ability to heal. Then I'd forget to have faith in the infinite possibilities and narrow my focus to the painful present. (You may be noticing a trend of forgetting and remembering, forgetting and remembering here.) One day I'd be filled with the hope and the will to heal; the next day doubt would cast its dark shadow on my every move. A little voice in my head kept saying, "What if you never walk again? What if you're destined for a life of chronic pain? What if this, right now, is as good as it gets?" This voice would follow me like my own personal raincloud, and when I tried to outrun it, I'd end up sliding backward in my recovery.

At the time, I was fortunate to have a partner who would often catch me underneath the shadow of doubt. With great confidence, my partner would exclaim, "You are going to walk again. You are going to get your life back. I just know it!" My partner was such a strong, sensitive, positive person, who held space for the belief in my recovery that I couldn't find within myself.

I decided at a certain point to use the phrase "in process" to describe my physical challenges. Eventually, through practice, I was able to hold onto my partner's vision for me for longer and longer stretches. The dark veil of doubt that had cast its ugly shadow on my life started to dissipate, giving rise to a visceral knowing in the depths of my soul. It became fully mine, this raw, unadulterated, potent knowing that I would fully recover. I still didn't know "how" or "when" I would heal, but I was certain that one day I'd resume normal functioning. I could picture myself walking along the beach below my apartment, my spine long, my hips level, my pain a distant memory. In my mind's eye, I could see myself free, freer than I'd ever been, my schedule cleared of the four arduous hours of rehab that took up every morning. Imagine what I could do with all that extra time! The vision was so clear, so divine, and it came with unshakable certainty. I would fully heal from this injury. I would get my life back. More than that, I would feel better than I'd ever felt in my life. I was going to come out of this on the other side as a more awakened human being.

Clarity of vision gave rise to a keen understanding that if I was in the flow of the river of life, the current would guide me to a complete recovery. In that flow, I could tap into the divine guidance all around me and listen deeply to my own healing intuition and inner wisdom. I was clearly able to see the infinite number of healing possibilities available to me at all times. Like a blind man who is miraculously able to see, I could now navigate my own healing process without my partner having to hold the vision for both of us.

From that point on things began to fall into place. A couple months after my first visit to St. James Cathedral, I had a joint appointment with my new physical therapist, Henry, who worked in conjunction with an orthopedic dentist. Dr. Molberly had spent the last twenty years crafting cutting-edge treatments to address chronic spine dysfunction from the top down, beginning with the jaw.

After going to hundreds of medical appointments over the last three years, this one wasn't all that different from the rest. What did feel different was a deep sense of gratitude that coursed through my heart. These two brilliant practitioners were so dedicated to helping me and all their other patients make the impossible possible. I felt a deep sense of love for both of them that stopped me in my tracks. That day, the three of us began collaborating, and they discovered a hitch in my system previously unrecognized. With that new information, they developed a new approach that would shape the course of my recovery, realigning my body one vertebra at a time.

As I began walking to my car, I noticed the nerve pain and numbness in my right leg was gone. My previously stuck left hip was moving normally again. I was walking freely, with grace and ease. Was I healed or at least closer to being healed? For the next few days, I could feel buzzy little pulses moving up and down my spine. It wasn't painful; rather, it felt like an electrical current was flowing within my spinal cord, like my nervous system was reorganizing itself from top to bottom. This brilliant reorganization paved the way for creation of new neural connections that would lead to unencumbered walking

Soon thereafter, I flushed my four pain medications down the toilet. My posture went from looking like a hunched-back ape to a ballerina. Virtually everywhere I went, people asked if I was a Pilates or yoga instructor. I stopped thinking of myself as a sick, frail person. I wasn't finished in my recovery process, but I'd taken a miraculous leap forward.

THE SPECIFICITY OF BELIEF

What is the difference between faith and belief? These two words are used interchangeably, or one is used to define the other and vice versa. Given how nebulous or personal the definitions may be, it makes sense that different people define and use them differently. I see them as subtly different from each other, yet each is essential in its own way.

In my mind, belief is more specific than faith and, to a degree, more intellectual. It's directional rather than open.

You believe in a specific treatment, a specific healer, or a specific outcome. It is a state of mind, a trust in something or someone. It's a potent form of internal knowing in which you know beyond a shadow of a doubt that you are headed toward a certain goal. Belief is not merely positive or wishful thinking, it's an inner knowing arising from the depths of your very being.

Let's return to that playground parachute metaphor. If falling with the knowledge that you will be safely caught is surrender, and the outward motion of being tossed in the air represents (positive) faith, then belief could be thought of as having a specific desire, like wanting to be thrown three feet in the air. You might even say to the people around you, "Hey everyone, last Tuesday you threw me 2.5 feet high. This week, let's go for three."

Essentially what this means is that you are turning an idea—in the form of a belief—into reality through intention and its resulting action. Having faith is the first step. For the publication of his book *Think and Grow Rich* in 1937, Napoleon Hill spent twenty-five years interviewing some of the world's richest men (at the time, it was only men), and found that faith was essential along with a belief, a vision. (That pioneering book is a great early reference for not just how to accumulate wealth but how to create a vision and then go about pursuing it.) Had easy printing of images and vision boards been invented then, I'm sure he would have been an avid proponent!

So what does this look like in real life? Let me tell you about my friend Becca who, at the age of forty-five, received a diagnosis of stage 4 breast cancer. Her doctor gently laid out the prognosis: the cancer could continue to spread. She could weaken to the point of incapacitation. There was a 70 percent chance she could die.

Obviously, this was very bad news. Like most sane people who have just received such a prognosis, she completely freaked out. She felt disappointed in the universe and sorry for herself and hopeless. She was a good person, wasn't she? She'd eaten kale and run three miles twice a week and drank purified water and went hiking in the woods every chance she got. She even filed her taxes early! In other words, she hadn't done everything right, but she'd done enough right to feel like she'd earned good health. Well, then why would she get such a horrible disease at such a young age? It wasn't fair.

Fortunately, Becca is not one to sit around being mad. So after a few days of shaking her fist at the sky, she took a long cold shower, brewed an extra-strong cup of coffee, and got busy.

In part, "busy" meant "deep introspection." She was able to recognize flailing and the fear behind it (an incredible feat), and when she felt the urge to *do* something rash, like ordering miracle pills off the Internet or burn all her bras, she would make herself sit down and take ten slow breaths. She started journaling every day with a focus on the cancer in her writing. As an intuition practice, she would ask herself questions regarding treatment before going to sleep. She began to regularly attend spiritual retreats to help her tap into her own healing energy through meditation. In the end, she underwent intensive hormone therapy and chemotherapy as well as an expansive array of healing modalities. A trusted naturopath helped her radically change her diet. An energy worker facilitated her work to address childhood trauma and release trapped emotions.

Now, five years cancer-free, Becca lives each day with great health, vitality, and enthusiasm. She took charge of her healing process and created a milieu of healing modalities to address mind, body and spirit.

The reason I'm telling this story is to illustrate some choices Becca made around faith and belief. The first choice she made was to have faith in the power of cancer and to believe in the prognosis as outlined by her oncologist. This was a possibility narrowed into a single dark tunnel leading toward decline and death. Had she stayed there, letting that choice pull her toward it, this would be a different story. Instead, she decided not to hold onto the original assumption that she would be a member of the 70 percent who die within five years and pivoted so that she assumed she would be a member of the 30 percent club, one of those who survived. Her doctor laid out those alternative scenarios of what life would look like while she sought treatment. With her oncologist's and medical team's support, Becca cultivated faith in her own power to heal, which led her to envision a cancer-free future and pursue an approach that she believed in and which did, in fact, lend itself to her healing.

I had a similar experience. I went from having absolute faith in my pain, in that I had faith that it would never go away, a feeling that was compounded by long sleepless nights. That negative faith led me to believe that suicide was my best option. Thank goodness my suicide attempt wasn't successful, and that healers entered my life just when I needed them. Because of their support, I was able to begin to have faith in my own power to heal, and from that I developed a belief system that turned an idea of being pain free into taking action to get there.

In order to even begin to see the infinite possibilities for healing, you have to believe beyond a shadow of a doubt that you will fully heal. Once the veil of doubt has been lifted, you can put up your radar for the guidance life will show you regarding what direction to head on your healing journey. The guidance you receive may not always make sense to the logical brain. For example, you may receive a signal guiding you to a non-traditional healing approach. Even if you can't see how it's all going to come together, the key is to stick to the vision and follow through, staying open to new possibilities. Don't let your logical mind talk you out of it. Your body is a brilliantly crafted system that knows what it needs to heal.

POSITIVITY AND POSSIBILITY

There are many stories of faith, belief, and miraculous healing. Then there are stories of delusion. How can you tell one from the other, positive belief from delusion? It would probably have made more sense for Becca to have believed in a negative outcome for her prognosis, yet none of us in her life thought she was being delusional when she chose to believe in the positive.

Popular culture has become obsessed with positive thinking over the last decade, from positive psychology to new age positive thinking paradigms. Thinking positive is more than great, it's essential for living a full, happy life. It's a wonderful idea to focus on creating positive thoughts and emotions in our lives. Let's all be about that! But a problem arises when we focus *solely* on the positive, thereby cutting ourselves off from or trying to outrun the negative.

Becca made a decision to focus on the positive but did not negate or deny the negative, did not delude herself into thinking that the chance of succumbing to cancer didn't exist. She knew very well that 70 percent of people with her diagnosis did not live past the five-year mark. Yet that did not stop her from doing what she could to improve her chances of survival. More importantly, she did not waste any energy on pretense.

If you've ever known anyone in full delusion mode, you know that it takes a tremendous amount of work for them to keep their head in the sand. Not that we can blame or shame anyone who goes this route—it is so, so hard to look pain, loss, and death square in the face. A friend of mine recently lost a child to cancer after a three-year-long struggle, and for much of that time she ardently refused to believe in the doctor's prognosis. Not for a second did it cross my mind for me to tell her to snap out of it and face reality. Ultimately, her child died despite her and their loved ones' faith and belief, and we could be tempted to call her belief delusion when we look at the eventual outcome. But for many people, even those who do not recover from cancer or paralysis or any number of diseases, their belief is what got them through the toughest moments and gave them a reason to live. It made them keep looking ahead, instead of resigning themselves to pain and death. In the end, wouldn't you rather lose after trying your best, rather than giving up from the start?

As Brene Brown points out, "We cannot selectively numb emotions. When we numb painful emotions, we also numb positive ones." Negative states compound if they're not properly addressed, and they are often the underlying cause of bad choices. What else is addiction and interpersonal violence but an explosive way to avoid dealing with an uncomfortable internal state? Then there's the flailing, my chosen method of active delusion. I can admit that I was in a delusional state right after my injury. I was in so much pain, alongside denial of that pain and my new circumstances. It's going to get better! I'd desperately tell myself, without a plan grounded in calm observation and patient data gathering, without really paying attention to what was actually happening. Desperation is the key word here—doing anything in a state of desperation is never a good idea. And so I'd rush off to my next appointment, and my next appointment, and the one after that.

Still, I'd highly recommend shifting off the "Why me?" and "It's never going to get better" mentality, the victimhood neural pathways that feed upon themselves and create depression, apathy, and inertia. I don't want to dismiss how hard things can be when you're not feeling well. As a psychotherapist, and as someone who knows this process all too well, I believe it's critical to work through any grief, frustration, anger, sadness with great compassion. What I am advocating, however, is that you can't afford to stay stuck on these negative pathways. From a neuroscience perspective, *where* we place our attention is *where* our brain develops. As Seghal et al. put it, "'Use it or lose it' is a popular adage often associated with use-dependent enhancement of cognitive abilities. Much research has focused on understanding exactly how the brain changes as a function of experience. Such experience-dependent plasticity involves both structural and functional alterations that contribute to adaptive behaviors, such as learning and memory, as well as maladaptive behaviors, including anxiety disorders, phobias, and posttraumatic stress disorder."[12] If you're focused on healing, if you're focused on infinite possibility, if you're focused on love, if you're focused on the gift of illness, injury, or trauma, then you're going to create healing and possibility pathways. By becoming obsessed with healing, love, and infinite possibilities, you have no other option but to generate these things within your life.

REFRAMING BELIEFS: NO PROBLEM

While focusing on the positive will help you generate a healing, it's essential that you don't use "positive thinking" to hide or bypass the difficulties that arise in your process. Instead, move toward and through these moments because in order to truly heal, we must make contact with all of our self, even the parts we don't like. As we turn toward our pain, facing what's difficult in our lives, we let love in. We engage with our difficulty, not forcefully or punitively, but with gentleness and patience. Part of shifting off negativity-focused pathways may involve working with a therapist or gifted healer. Working through the difficult emotions that accompany any healing process is absolutely necessary in order for you to begin to reclaim your health. With help or on our own, as we give ourselves to our struggle, we become the answer to our struggle. By responding to our lives from a healthy, connected place, we become the answer to our greatest problems. The wisdom inside of us becomes alive and guides us toward greater truth and healing. As J. Krishnamurti said, "It's the truth that liberates, not your effort to be free." True healing always involves making contact with all of ourselves, finding the light within amidst the lingering darkness, while being held in a container love and support.

So how do we change our beliefs without falling into the delusion trap? We look at the problem full in the face and then place it within its context. Life isn't over until it's over and, despite how it might feel in the moment, this problem is not permanent. To paraphrase what the Greek philosopher Heraclitus said 2,500 years ago, as so many other people have done: "The only constant is change."

You can think about it like this: If you can expand your awareness around the problem, there is no problem. How do you expand your awareness around the problem? Change your perception. You can do this by using the "3 No Problems" process. Simply think about the challenge and reframe it by reminding yourself:

- It's not a problem, it's a starting point.
- It's not a problem, it's a decision that needs to be made.
- It's not a problem, it's a call to action.

I used the "3 No Problems" process throughout my rehabilitation, especially during the times when I felt stuck or overwhelmed. At a certain point, for example, I'd stopped making progress with a gifted physical therapist who had helped me out of the abyss of acute pain. I was terrified to work with anyone else, but something needed to change. Using the "3 No Problems," first I looked at the conundrum with my physical therapist as a starting point. Was it a problem, or was it actually an opportunity to find another gifted healer who could help me navigate the next leg of my journey? Second, I realized that it was time to make a decision to start seeing another PT. Third, I took ownership of the direction that I needed to head in and began to take action.

When I thought hard about it, I could recognize that there was nothing wrong in the universe, and life wasn't against me. Rather, life was asking me to step up to the plate, to expand my awareness around the problem in order to allow for a new possibility. In doing so, I connected with a new physical therapist with whom I had miraculous results.

You can change your beliefs without denying reality by placing them within their rightful context. Take charge of your situation, knowing that everything is exactly as it should be in this moment and the universe is always in your court.

THE SCIENCE OF BELIEF

The most powerful treatment for any ailment is stimulating the body to heal itself. I was introduced to this concept in 1998 as a clinical psychology graduate student at the University of Washington. Since then, there have been thousands of brilliantly designed studies with findings that have demonstrated that positive belief alone can alleviate symptoms and heal the body. This mystical interplay between mind, body, and belief is also known as the placebo effect.

The placebo effect is more than positive thinking—it's believing a treatment or procedure will work. It's located in the connection between the brain and body and how they work together. In essence, the placebo effect is evidence that positive belief can alleviate symptoms and heal the body.

While more research is needed to understand the healing relationship of the mind/body connection, we can look to an array of research studies that demonstrate how belief influences healing of the body, even in the presence of great pain and dysfunction. Dr. Bruce Moseley, an orthopedic surgeon known for healing people with debilitating knee pain, designed a controlled clinical study (J. Bruce Moseley et al., 2011) in which one group of patients received surgery while the other group underwent an extravagantly crafted phony surgery.

During the fake surgery, the patients were sedated, given three small incisions, and shown a prerecorded tape of someone else's procedure on the video monitor. The doctors and nurses even splashed water around to mimic the sound of a procedure.

The findings were that knee pain of one-third of the patients who received the real surgery were resolved. No surprise there. What shocked the researchers, however, was that the people who received the fake surgery got the same resolution of knee pain. At a certain point in the study, the participants receiving the fake surgery had a *greater* reduction in pain than those who actually received the real surgery!

Published in the *New England Journal of Medicine*, one of the most highly respected medical journals worldwide, this study was randomized and double-blind, and it showed a significant percentage of patients experiencing a remission of their knee pain because they believed they received surgery.

The mind can be a powerful healing tool when given the chance. The idea that your brain can convince your body a fake treatment is the real thing—the placebo effect—and thus stimulate healing has been around for millennia. Religious and cultural rituals around healing, from "faith healings" to moon ceremonies to oil dripping to reiki, endure because they have worked for many people for many years. Choosing a healing course and a trustworthy practitioner, with an attitude of "I'm all in," allows for the mystical interplay of mind, body, and the healing process to unfold. When you are making this choice around a modality or a practitioner, however, check in with your internal GPS.

Reflection Questions

I'd like to invite you to take a deep breath and answer the following questions as honestly as possible.

- What are your current beliefs around illness, injury, and trauma?
- What are your beliefs around healing?
- Can you tell the difference between belief and delusion? Are the choices you are making more inspired by fear or hope?
- What "problem" could benefit from a reframing of perception?
- Do you trust the practitioners and the healing modalities that they offer?
- Are you simpatico in the way you and the practitioner(s) view illness, injury, and trauma?
- How does the practitioner assess you and your body? Is it holistic or more focused? (Neither way is the "right" way, but you want to make sure you understand their angle.)
- Does the practitioner seem genuine, caring, forthright? Is your practitioner open, attentive, controlling, rigid, knowledgeable, curious?
- Do the practitioners take pride in their ability to heal others, or do they take pride in their ability to facilitate others' self-healing?
- Does the practitioner have your best interests at heart?
- How does the service or plan build on other ways in which you are healing yourself? How does it fit into the larger picture in terms of your health and wellness?

CHAPTER 6

The Mystical Power of Embodied Imagination

"You must find the place inside yourself where nothing is impossible."—Deepak K. Chopra

A few years ago a friend of mine invited me over for dinner. With bottle of wine in hand, I knocked on the door of his Madison Valley town house overlooking Lake Washington. "Kat!" he said with a smile after opening the door. "Come on in."

I stepped inside, and what I saw took my breath away. There, plastered to the walls and the refrigerator, the countertop and the kitchen table, even the television, were hundreds of sticky notes. I took off my shoes, handed him the wine, and peered closely at one of the little yellow papers next to the wall by the front door. "I am in love with my soulmate," it said in all caps. I took a step to the left. "My soulmate is strongly attracted to me," said the next. Above that one said, "I will manifest the most loving person in my life." The rest followed in this vein: "I am a magnet attracting my perfect partner now" and "My heart is open" and "Destiny brings my soulmate and I together" and "I am love" and so on.

"Looks like you're looking for love," I said, stating the obvious.

"Yup," he confirmed, moving into the kitchen and taking a wine key out of a drawer. He popped the cork, poured a glass, and handed it to me, then poured one for himself. "Dinner's about fifteen minutes away," he said. The scent of garlic and onions filled the air, making my mouth water. "In the meantime, let's sit and enjoy our wine," he said.

At the kitchen table, I took a sip and asked, "So, what are you looking for?"

"Oh, you know. Someone who is smart and funny and pretty and kind," he replied.

"Sure," I said. "Aren't we all. How's the search going?"

"Terrible, honestly. I've been on like a thousand dates, and they're all the same. We meet for coffee or a drink, make small talk, and then she ghosts me. It happens like that every time. I guess no one wants to be with me," he said. With his words, the energy in the room shifted. There we were, surrounded by brightly colored squares of paper on nearly every available surface, yet the mood was dark. Clearly he was disappointed in his love life and held hostage to feelings of worthlessness. The rainbow of positive affirmations had yet to do its job of making him feel positive and affirmed in himself and his desire. Needless to say, his attempts to attract his soul mate had not yet been successful.

WALKING THE WALK

Remember the difference between delusion and belief? Belief is a potent knowing grounded in an acknowledgement of reality as it is and a simultaneous vision for the future. Delusion, on the other hand, generally takes the form of flailing and is driven by fear, grasping, and desperation. With the utmost respect to my friend and his situation, I have to say honestly that putting hundreds of Post-it notes on the walls doesn't look good in the desperation department. Can you imagine going to a potential love interest's house and seeing that? I don't know about you, but I'd run screaming in the other direction. On top of that, his emotional state did not match the words he'd written. "My heart is open" is just not a powerful statement when you are downcast, despairing, and focused on past rejection. His body language conveyed the opposite of openheartedness—when he talked about his love life, he slouched, his shoulders rolling forward and his chest sinking. That, and the disparity between the written words "Destiny brings my soulmate and I together" and the spoken words "I guess no one wants to be with me," was just too strong.

Essentially, those words were empty because of a mismatch between them and the actual feeling, the emotion versus thought, intention, and/or action. He *wanted* love; his intention was to find love, but he did not *feel* love. He did not *have* love, not really, and he was not actively *being* love. And it's really hard, if not impossible, to create something from nothing.

I don't blame my friend for feeling despair and dejection. Anyone who didn't meet the love of their life in high school is likely familiar with the toll a string of bad dates and bad partners can take on the heart, the self-esteem, the soul, the checkbook, the faith in humanity. Still, I can only assume that his dating behavior was not aligned with the spirit of love, but rather took the form, however subtle, of neediness or dejectedness or self-protectiveness.

After a delicious meal and another glass of wine, my friend admitted that he tended to either come on a little strong or be almost completely passive, depending on what kind of hit his pride had taken on his previous adventure in dating. He would invite someone over too soon, or text too frequently or with too many emojis. (Some advice for you singles out there: one emoji is great, two is fine, three is iffy, and four is creepy. Also, one exclamation point does the trick. And please, for the love of all that is holy, wait a goodly long time before sending a pic of yourself without clothes on!) Sometimes, he'd go in for a kiss simply because it was the end of the date, without assessing body language or asking permission. Other times, he would just not follow up after a night out with someone, no matter how well it went, because he assumed that the woman was too smart or too funny or too pretty or too kind to ever be interested in a loser like him.

My friend was talking the talk via a million Post-it notes but not walking the walk, and anyone with half a brain could tell. In this way, his outer world and inner world were actually perfectly aligned, in that his feelings of hopelessness and worthlessness were causing certain behaviors, which repelled women like a bad smell which, in turn, fed into his feelings of hopelessness and worthlessness, which caused certain behaviors, and so the cycle went round and round. The time and energy he'd put into plastering every available surface with positive affirmations, of essentially putting a hundred brightly covered Band-Aids over a festering emotional wound, he could have been using to address his inner space, to examine his true feelings (and his true woundings) and how they impacted his behaviors.

The process of writing mantras like "I am love" and "My perfect partner is on her way" can be a practice of auto-suggestion, whereby you eventually train your mind away from negative self talk and toward a desired narrative or set of beliefs. There is something to faking it until you make it, in the sense that you practice over and over and over again who you want to be until you become that person. But, at the time of our dinner together, he was still too enthralled in negative narratives with too much faith in loneliness and rejection. Perhaps, in time, he would come to internalize the messages on those Post-it notes, which would result in him behaving in ways that aligned with an intention of love, which would attract a loving partner. But in that moment he still had a long way to go.

CO-CREATING WITH THE UNIVERSE

There's nothing magical about the idea that your inner world impacts the outer world, and the outer world impacts your inner world and that, at the end of the day, the line between outer and inner is an illusion. We—plants, animals, minerals, the stars, the dirt, electricity, chemistry, biology—are all connected in this crazy web of life. While you or I might see a cute little meadow mushroom poking its round cap out of the lawn, what we can't see is the vast connection between what seems to be an individual (but actually isn't) and the rest of the world through the mycelium network. Same goes for many kinds of trees via what some clever scientist dubbed the "wood wide web." And humans, too, of course, though we don't have a root structure that hooks us up to one another belowground. We may feel separate, but we truly share everything, from oxygen to air-borne viruses, language to the impulses that make up human nature to the stories, rituals, cuisines, color schemes, and moral tenets that make up culture. Then there's the *world* wide web—what else is a meme but an idea connecting ten people or twenty people or two million people on the Internet? What is money but a shared belief that little green slips of paper and little rectangles of plastic and numbers on a computer screen have value? What is society but a shared agreement to a standard set of rules?

To experience how we are all connected, all you have to do is walk down the street. The sight of someone passed out drunk changes your mood, doesn't it? As an empath, my mood is very easily influenced—spotting a couple arguing on the street, or watching a news story about a school shooting, or even experiencing an extended period of gray weather can tug my mood downward if I'm not paying attention. At the same time, a stranger giving me a big bright smile as they walk by can light up my day.

I might be on the more extreme side of the empathy spectrum, but most neurotypical people experience the same emotional connectivity to some degree. It's multi-directional—if you get a little ping of joy when a stranger smiles at you, you'll probably feel a similar ping when you smile at a stranger. Your mood has the power to change your behavior, your behavior has the power to change your mood, and you have the power to impact the mood and behaviors of those around you; to change both their outer and inner worlds.

All this is to say that we share the world, that no part of us is separate from any other part, and that reality responds to our thoughts and feelings and vice versa. The thoughts and feelings that make up your inner world affect your behavior, which affects the way you imprint yourself on the world, which in turn, affects the way the world treats you.

Not everyone recognizes this fairly simple interplay, or knows how to use it to advantage. Oftentimes, when we're faced with challenging circumstances, we tend to feel discouraged or even helpless. We may feel like victims of our own destiny, that life is not happening for us, it's happening to us. The critical thing to understand is that we are both players on the game board of life, *and* we are the game board of life. We are part of the network, *and* we are the network. Life is not "happening" to us but rather, we are life.

This shift in perception changes everything.

Your current situation is one possibility in reality, but it's certainly not the only one. Your situation is not a fixed entity. There are, in fact, many possibilities when it comes to reality, and as you grow in your healing practices, you gain more and more power to dramatically alter the course of your life and to become fully engaged in the web of life.

There are people who, no matter the hand they were dealt, have overcome all odds and learned how to rise above their circumstances. There are a million and one examples: the woman born into poverty who earns a college scholarship and goes on to become a successful entrepreneur; the man who, as a child, suffered abuse at the hands of his parents and yet goes on to become a loving father. All the people born into a society that systemically oppressed them but somehow came to believe that they deserved better and so fought for it. How did they do that? Mind over matter.

Mind over matter is the ability to transcend the limitations that hinder us from reaching our full potential by using the power of the mind. Before the woman who became a successful entrepreneur could take a single step away from the poverty she grew up in, she had to understand that there were options besides poverty. She had to believe in her power to work hard and succeed and then make a plan and take action. Before the man who became a loving father could take a single step away from the abuse he'd suffered, he had to understand that there were parenting styles different from the kind he'd experienced. He had to believe in his power to form healthy, loving relationships and make a plan for how to be a better father than the one he'd had and take action. The seeds of change began in their minds.

We could also say that the seeds of change began in their hearts. What was it that got them interested in figuring out a different way to live in the first place? Perhaps it was a caring aunt or a teacher who went above and beyond the call of duty and gave them a glimpse of an alternative reality. Perhaps it was a good book or television show that awakened them to the fact that their current circumstances weren't the only circumstances available. Whatever it was that gave them this insight, it wasn't just cold hard facts that sparked desire to make change; it was hope, an elevated energy, that sparked desire as well. The combination of elevated energy, intention, and a solid plan is just about unstoppable.

To co-create with the universe, you must understand that the energy you're emitting into the universe is the same energy you receive back. The joy that brings about a smile elicits a smile; the irritability that brings about a frown elicits a frown. The greed that compels you to steal from the till brings about retribution, expulsion, jail time. The generosity that compels you to deliver hot soup to a sick friend brings about hot soup from a friend when you need it. In short, you reap what you sow. Truly, each of us has the opportunity to influence our reality through a combination of thought, intention, and emotion. Or, in other words, "embodied imagination."

EMBODIED IMAGINATION

As a lifelong Seattlelite, I'm accustomed to five to eight months of rain every year. Like many locals, by the time March rolls around, I'm pale, exhausted, and somewhat depressed from the lack of sunlight. Of course, there are physiological elements at play, like the very really effects of vitamin D deficiency. That, at least, is an easy fix—just get yourself down to a natural grocery store or chain drug store and buy a vitamin D supplement.

What else can you do in the middle of January when you can't even remember what blue sky looks like? Praying for sun is all well and good, but that is not the most reliable method for making the clouds go away because, well, clouds do what they want, when they want. I just don't think we can control the weather, beyond moving somewhere with a climate more to our liking. What we can control is our internal weather. We can let the sun shine on the inside.

Take a moment now and close your eyes and begin to feel a feeling as though the sun has already arrived. Feel the feeling of the warm rays on your skin, of every muscle in your body loosening and relaxing. Feel the feeling of tranquility as you bask in the warmth. Feel the feelings of your bare feet on the warm grass, the green blades soft beneath you.

When you pause and put your attention on creating feelings, you can actually feel them, can't you? You can alter your internal state without waiting for the sun to actually show its face. The brain is a magical machine, and when you imagine that the sun is here, then, in your body, it is.

Scientific research has shown that when we feel a feeling of love, compassion, understanding, or forgiveness, we change our self-esteem. According to research done by Rollin McCraty of the HeartMath Research Center, the change in self-esteem has an effect on the electrical and magnetic fields in the heart. (McCraty, 2019) Because what is a feeling but a combination of chemistry, biology, electricity? What is a feeling but the seed of impulse that leads to action?

For my friend who wanted to attract his perfect partner, it would therefore make sense to live as though his perfect partner has already arrived, to cultivate a feeling of love, both the receiving and the giving of it. He would imagine what it would feel like to wake up next to his soul mate, what it would feel like to support and accept his soul mate, what it would feel like to wash dishes together and take long walks on a beach together and build a life together. If he imagined that scenario in which his soul mate had arrived and embodied the feeling of love, that would certainly impact the choices he made, how he chose to spend his time, and how he chose to present himself to the world. I imagine that if he went on dates already feeling love, versus grasping or running away, he'd be a much more appealing candidate.

This is how you fulfill desire: you imagine, in your body, the feeling of your desire already being fulfilled.

I experienced the extraordinary results of embodied imagination firsthand. About three years into my healing journey, I was reflecting upon my sole intention: to walk normally in the absence of pain. I'd been through so many different therapies, all of which focused on muscle activation, pain reduction, and autonomic nervous regulation, all without much success. I treated my rehab like a job, the kind that's a grind and not a joy. I'd spent thousands of hours in physical therapy, doing at least five-hundred different exercises that in all honesty didn't do much. I religiously practiced walking for two or three hours a day. In total, I spent seven hours every day to get myself moving.

I'd begun to realize that those therapies would only take me so far, and in pursuit of self-healing, I looked into books and articles about people who had healed themselves by using a combination of intention and elevated emotion. *Mind to Matter: The Astonishing Science of How Your Brain Creates Material Reality* by Dawson Church, *Breaking the Habit of Being Yourself* by Joe Dispenza, *Quantum Healing: Exploring the Frontiers of Mind/Body Medicine* by Deepak Chopra, *The Science Of Miracles: The Quantum Language of Healing, Peace, Feeling, and Belief* by Gregg Braden, and *Radical Remission: Surviving Cancer Against All Odds* by Kelly A. Turner were a few that changed my mind.

If the people in these books could do it, so could I! Now, every morning before I got out of bed, I guided myself through a 10-minute mind/body exercise, feeling the feeling of being able to wake up in the morning and move into the world with grace and ease. I felt the feeling of fluidity and freedom, as every muscle in my body relaxed. I envisioned myself walking along the beach, my head held high, my back straight, my stride strong. I *felt* what that felt like, from an internal perspective. I would feel the sensation of my feet in the sand, my even steps, my chest open, the fresh wind blowing on my face. I felt what it was like to walk not just without pain but with strength, joy and grace.

This was not a magical cure but rather a slow internal process of inviting new possibilities for movement into my life. Prior to engaging in this practice, I would wake up already grumpy and frustrated, negative feelings that spilled over into my day. Whenever I left the house, I'd been focused on the strain in my step and paranoid that random people on the street were staring at me as I limped by. The belief in other's judgments had made it so I became even more self conscious, which caused me to clam up, which caused my limp to get worse, which probably increased the likelihood of drawing curious stares. At a certain point, I didn't want to leave the house, and in my isolation, I became stuck in a negative feedback loop. That's how my life was for almost three years: narrow. The thing is, that once I started to have faith in healing, to believe in the healing practices I was doing and the practitioners I was seeing, to have a vision for the future, and to embody that future as though it was here now, my stride changed. And so my confidence changed, like a toddler who, after hours of practice, can go for a stretch of teeter-totter walking without falling on her behind.

On the third year anniversary of my injury, I mediated all morning before my intuition guided me to visit the spot where I had been injured. Enveloped in a deep sense of peace, balance, and equanimity, I headed down the long stretch of sandy beach, then dropped to my knees in the sand. With gratitude I surrendered to the divine, and I again began to visualize myself walking normally and without pain. Because I'd practiced so much, every part of my being could sense what this moment would feel like. Once the felt sense of walking was imprinted in every cell of my body, I set a clear intention, using the advice of a Peruvian Shaman healer for how to word it:

> *"May the Universe and I co-create walking in a way that is peaceful, with ease, kindness to myself, the world and others, and serves the higher good of all."*

I again visualized myself walking once more with grace and ease. I again felt the feelings of being able to move freely and fluidly. Then I let go so the universe could do its work.

I continued to walk the Washington Park Arboretum over and over again, watching the cycles of the trees and flowers on safe ground, able to appreciate some of the beauty but still distracted by my awkward gait. Yet as my confidence increased, I started taking little detours to nearby coffeeshops, where I'd write and, every now and then, get into conversation with new people. At this point, a friend I'd met at a meditation retreat invited me to meet her at the farmer's market. This would mean crowds and unfamiliar terrain, but I felt ready for the challenge. I'd become less afraid of other's stares and so, if they were even bothering to look at me, I didn't notice. After that successful outing, my world continued to expand. I went out with old friends and new ones, to music concerts and different parks around the city. I even went on a day trip to Whidbey Island, taking the ferry across the wide blue Puget Sound. On the deck, the fresh wind blew across my face, just as I'd imagined.

Once I stopped envisioning myself as a frail person and stopped feeling like a sick person, and instead started envisioning and feeling healthy and vital, my life in the inner world got bigger and bigger, my life in the outer world got bigger and bigger, and a new cycle began. My old identity let go of its tight grip and a new identity took its place; one in which I accepted myself as I was and had endless hope for the future. Gratitude filled my heart.

When you create a state of being in your body, you begin to create that future event in the present moment. Change starts from within.

Steps to Co-Creating with the Universe

1. Become clear and specific about your new intention.
2. Without judging the old possibility, invite a new possibility into your life. Ask, "May we, the Universe and I, co-create [your desire] in a way that has peace, ease, kindness to self, world and others, and serves the higher good of all."
3. Feel the feelings of what your life would be like if the new possibility had already arrived.
4. Begin to live every day as if the new possibility has already happened.
5. Surrender your ego and trust the divine intelligence of the universe.
6. Be receptive to signs and listen to your intuition.
7. Give thanks to the new possibility as if it had already arrived.

Reflection Questions

I'd like to invite you to take a deep breath and answer the following questions as honestly as possible.

- What are some the feelings that primarily occupy your attention? Do you tend toward feelings of anger, helplessness, dejection? Do you tend toward acceptance, appreciation, hope?

- How do you experience the world? How does the world treat you?
- In what ways does your inner world match your outer world? In what ways are your inner world and outer world misaligned? In what ways are you talking the talk but not walking the walk?
- Do you believe you have the power to change your inner world? Do you believe you have the power to change your outer world?
- What is it you want? Does your inner world align with that desire? If so, how? If not, how?
- What are you doing in your outer world to get what you want? How are you choosing to live?

CHAPTER 7

Healing for Each Other

"Most people need love and acceptance a lot more than they need advice."—John Gottman

The day before had been dark, dreary, and depressing. I was in a phase where I was making real progress, and I could even accept those off days; days when I had pain or backslid in my recovery. Healing is not a linear process, nor is it an evenly sloped upward line on a tidy little graph. Every day is different.

The thing that had bummed me out on that particular day was not pain or a loss of mobility, but it was a series of conversations that had gotten me down. Per usual, I'd woken up early and trudged to the gym, where I spent an hour or two limping from one strength-training machine to the next. Most everyone there knew me as well as my story and had seen me do similar workout routines over the past few years. For whatever reason, that day everyone seemed to want to give me simplistic and unsolicited advice for how to best to deal with a very complex problem, one that they had witnessed me diligently working on for all that time. I'd been amazed at how quick acquaintances were to offer their opinions, suggestions, or even, in some cases, armchair diagnoses.

"You need to get on with your life," one very unhelpful person told me. *Okay,* I thought, *that's vague.*

"You can't let this injury become your identity," someone else said.

Yup, I thought. *But you try not internalizing years of experience!*

"There is this self-help book you should read," a guy at the grocery store explained.

I read that book a million years ago, I thought.

"You are too young to be having these kind of problems," said a well-intentioned older friend of a friend.

That's one million percent less than helpful, I thought.

These conversations drew me deeper and deeper into the dark abyss that I'd spent so much blood, sweat, and tears crawling out of. At least now I had the tools not to go into panic mode. These comments would not send me off into a binge of flailing. I'd long ago let go of my coping method of work, work, work, technology, exercise, and more work so that at the end of what felt like a very bad day, I sat with the emotional pain, frustration and anger. *How dare they tell me what to do!* I thought self-righteously. *Don't they know how hard I've been working! They have no idea what it's like to be me!*

There is a quote from *The Tibetan Book of the Living and Dying* that had helped me many times over the years, and I brought it to mind now, to help me reflect and calm down: "Whatever you do, don't try and escape your pain, but be with it. Because the attempt to escape from pain creates more of it."

That night, I met up with Laura, a friend I'd seen regularly for the past five years or so. We'd met through our graduate school program and initially bonded over our interest in clinical psychology and the amount of stress our studies were giving us. For the first couple years of our relationship, we'd get together over tea or a meal, and commiserate about our various difficulties, how it was impossible to get support, and how we felt burned out. Her understanding and sympathy were invaluable to me during a time when I was struggling and couldn't see a way out.

When I'd gotten injured, she'd been there for me, happy to listen to my complaints and to list some of her own. Suffering was the glue that bonded us.

That evening after the unsolicited advice spree of all those acquaintances and strangers, we met at a local organic restaurant. Over turmeric yam soup, kale salad, and kombucha, I told her about my day. "Those assholes!" she said. "God, people are so terrible sometimes." She then went on to tell me at great length about an interaction she'd had earlier that day, in which some jerk at work had had asked her to watch her tone and said that it would make their work together easier if she would be a little less harsh. "Whatever," she said to me. "Next thing you know, she'll be telling me I should smile more." She took a bite of her salad. "Being nice is not my job," she added.

Suddenly I realized how much our friendship was based on these kinds of mutual rantings. Laura believed that she had more than her fair share of things to complain about; that everyone else was incompetent or lazy and conflict was always someone else's fault. This was not a comfortable realization for me—I was so grateful for all the ways in which she had been there for me during the past five years. Yet now that I was trying to let go of a sense of victimhood, to claim responsibility for my life and for my own power to create it as I wished, I had to recognize that perhaps our attitudes and goals no longer aligned. *I love her*, I thought. *But is this the kind of person I want to spend my time with?*

The following day I woke up at the usual hour. From the moment I opened my eyes, I was wrestling with the same dark thoughts left over from the previous day, but I was also able to stay open to the idea of letting some light in should it come my way. I got dressed, drank a cup of coffee, and headed off to gym to begin my regiment of stretches and exercises. The day was gray, yet every now and then a crack of blue sky peaked through the clouds.

At the gym, I ran into my good friend Susan, a nurse who worked at Swedish Hospital and had beautiful long gray hair, a carefree attitude, and her own personal experience with pain.

"How are you?" she asked.

For a second, I considered answering politely with "fine" or "good, how are you?" Instead, I answered her honestly. "You know, I'm having a hard day," I said. "Yesterday I ran into a bunch of people who all seemed to have an opinion about my situation, without even really knowing me. They all had a suggestion for how to fix me. And then I had dinner with this old friend who is just plain angry at the world."

After a couple minutes of patiently listening to me vent my frustrations, Susan looked into my eyes. I paused. She took a deep breath, holding space for me to be right where it was, with all my pain, baggage, imperfections, and injured body parts. There was simply love and acceptance. Finally, she said, "The only thing you need right now is love."

In that moment, a sense of peace flowed through me. Here was someone who did not try to match me complaint for complaint, who sympathized without getting roped into negativity. She'd heard me out, truly listened, then pointed me toward love.

I thanked her, and we said our goodbyes, then I trekked down to the pool only to find that every lane was full. My swimming exercises were very important to me, but I usually dreaded swimming when it was so crowded, because sometimes I'd get kicked in the side or hit in the face by the other swimmers. Sometimes people would get annoyed with my slower pace. But that day, I felt like I was swimming with angels. The love that Susan had given me had filled me up, had spread into every cell of my body, and with that, I could see the world through that same nonjudgmental, wholly accepting filter. As I submerged my head under the water and gazed across the lanes through the lenses of my goggles, the swimmers appeared as though under a giant ray of light, their movements filled with a divine grace, their bodies beauty in motion.

Everything became so clear under the water. Love is how we sit with our pain. Love is how we heal. By allowing ourselves to be held by others and receive love, we can move through it and come out the other side. Through that, we can learn to love ourselves. Most important of all, we learn to give love in return.

CHOOSING YOUR TRIBE

The healing journey is a transformative process that involves continuous growth and transition, an ascension into one's higher purpose. This is an incredible gift of injury, illness, and trauma: it pushes you to examine and claim responsibility for yourself and your life. Most people are not the same going in as they are coming out, and as you evolve, so too will many of your relationships.

We are tribal creatures by nature. We build strong bonds that often endure through thick and thin. A healthy tribe allows you to have freedom for personal growth while acting as a secure base to which you can come home. It is this mix of freedom and attachment that allows you to reach your highest potential.

Other tribes or tribe members, however, may be threatened or simply unsupportive of your personal growth process. Relationships with these people or groups aren't necessary "bad" or "toxic." Rather, they drain you rather than fill you, deplete rather than nourish. Remaining in these relationships pose the danger of stunting your growth.

Just as your tribe in the real world has the potential to hurt, hinder, or heal, these days we have to consider social media its own kind of tribe because for many, it is the manifestation of the confusion between real and unreal. The age of technology has hit us by storm, and only time will tell what the long-term impacts will be. In the short term, it distracts us from the present moment in that we are constantly looking down at our devices rather than at each other directly, and it puts us in a chronic state of reactivity, seduced by instant gratification and fake connection. As a result, we've become disconnected from ourselves and from each other. On a large scale, our technology obsession has led to a pandemic of loneliness. A 2010 meta-analytic review of studies that examined the correspondence of social isolation and mortality showed that out of more than 300,000 people worldwide, those with strong relationships were 50 percent less likely to die in a given time frame.[13] In fact, research has shown that loneliness is even worse for longevity than being obese or physically inactive.

> *"No other factor in medicine, not smoking, not exercise, not stress, not genetics, not drugs or surgery affects our health, quality and length of life more than feeling loved and cared for."—* *Dean Ornish*

We can look at this another way. Social connection has been proven to be more beneficial than abstaining from drinking and smoking, or the presence of a good diet and exercise.[14]

This tells us that on average, those who live, eat, and rest with others live longer even if they eat unhealthy food, drink alcohol, smoke, or don't exercise. This effect can be seen in Denmark, Norway, Sweden and Switzerland, countries with cultures that value a lifestyle based on social connection and time spent relaxing. They also hold the top statistics on health and well-being in the world (Trimble, 2018)

These findings illustrate how vital the right kind of human connection is, not only to our health and wellbeing, but in many cases to our very lives. Unfortunately, there are no substitutes for real human interaction. One of the biggest obstacles to stepping away from technology is the belief that everyone else is online and that in order to have social interaction, you must be online too. This is absolutely not true. While many people are indeed online, countless others are not.

Another obstacle is the addictive high technology gives us. Have you ever received a bunch of likes on a post on Facebook, Instagram, or Twitter? Feels good, right? Those are your dopamine pathways (your feel-good brain chemicals) at work. Like with cigarettes and alcohol, many develop an insensitivity to this dopamine hit, requiring them to post more and vie for more *likes* in pursuit of the next and bigger hit. Fifteen *likes* might have felt good yesterday, but today no less than twenty will do, and if you don't get a hundred tomorrow, then the whole day was a waste. This need for digital validation can compel you to present an image that might be greatly skewed from reality. Don't believe what you see on social media—whether it's someone else's perfect Hawaiian vacation or your own.

Technology is a wonderful tool if used with intention. Having an infinitude of information at your fingertips can be an incredible blessing (if you know how to tell the true from the false). It can introduce you to new people with whom you wouldn't otherwise come in contact. How many friendships and business partnerships started in online networking forums? How many marriages have sprung from online dating sites? Of course, you have to look up from your phone, tie your shoes, and go out in the real world to make real connections.

It is there, in the real world, where you might realize that it's time to leave a relationship or a tribe. Chances are if you are recognizing a relationship's endpoint, it's not a good fit on either side and staying in can be harmful to all involved. That doesn't make it any easier—at the end is often when we cling the tightest. Change is hard, and if you're already in the process of big change, every additional change can be additionally difficult. Part of it comes down to routine. Giving up the monthly dinner date with the friend who spends all your time together complaining and blaming leaves wide open one night a month. Breaking up with a significant other who you love but don't trust is incredibly painful and can leave a hole in your heart. And then there's family. What to do about the overly critical parent, the passive-aggressive sibling, the friendly uncle who only pays a visit when he needs a favor? For family, there's no easy answer (though there are many books about how to set healthy boundaries).

Building your life with intentionality requires all of your energy, and so you have to decide whether you will carry the weight of someone who brings you down or gets in your way, or if you will let them go. Whatever your decision, I recommend that you approach them with kindness, honesty, and sincerity. Sometimes the simple act of calling out a harmful pattern can open up a conversation that leads to a new style of relating. Then you can keep that relationship. If not, well, then maybe it's time to let it go.

I had to look at my friendship with Laura and decide whether it was worth saving. Ultimately, after a couple of rough conversations, we concluded that we were no longer on the same page. It was painful but in the end, it was the right decision. I was creating a new life for myself, and I needed a tribe that aligned with my daily practice of positive faith and pursuit of higher purpose.

This waking up can force you out of some of your current relationships and into the unknown. This is the normal, natural progression, and it will shake your very foundation. I have found, however, that when I leave one relationship, the universe brings a new one that's more aligned with who I am in the moment and who I aspire to be. The rule of thumb is: You have to let go of the old to make space for the new to arise. Always do so with kindness.

Each person achieves the creation of new connections in different ways. Some people more actively surround themselves with family and friends. Others join a support group, exercise class, or spiritual group where they can connect with likeminded peers or people working through a similar healing process. Some people feel most connected when they are alone, through prayer, mediation, writing, or making art.

At some juncture in your healing journey, you will move from survive mode to thrive mode. Relationship and connection are inextricably part of this growth process. As you begin to grow and transform, so will your relationships.

RELATIONSHIPS THAT NOURISH AND SUSTAIN

Not all relationships are created equal. Every unique connection has its own pulse that leaves us feeling fulfilled, neutral, or depleted. After getting together with my lifelong best friend, I feel deeply nourished, like I've eaten a hamburger big and juicy enough to sustain me for month. After spending time with an acquaintance named Jim, who is perfectly nice but with whom I don't share many interests, I'm left feeling hungry, like I've eaten a single rice cracker. And then there is Grace—after hanging out with her, I feel like I've eaten week-old sushi.

Of course, we can't be around only those people who nourish and sustain us all of the time. We all have to deal with people with whom we just don't get, or who don't get us. That's just part of living in the world. When you're digging your way out of a difficult situation, however, the company you keep is vital to your success. Be aware of how much time you are willing to spend with people who bring you down, take more then they give, waste your time, pull you backward, or have no authentic interest in you. While it will be impossible to avoid these types of people altogether, at the very least you can choose to not allow them to drain your energy.

You decide how you want to invest your time and energy, how you want to attract those who love, inspire, and fulfill you, and for whom you can do the same. There's no reason to settle for less, at least not within your closest circle.

So what does a healthy, loving relationship feel like?

- Both sides feel seen and heard by the other.
- Both sides communicate and listen with compassion.
- Both sides genuinely care for the other.
- Both sides show up consistently and authentically.
- Both sides are congruent in their words and their actions.
- Both sides feel met and matched by the other.

Note here that I wrote "both sides." Illness, injury, and trauma can cause a survival-motivated selfishness, and that's OK. In fact, not only is it OK, it is essential to ask for help and receive the help that's given when in crisis.

For much of this book, we've been examining methods by which we can reclaim our power to heal ourselves. This is an essential process, yet healing is never a solitary endeavor. We are a social species by nature, wired for love and connection in our very DNA. To think that we could possibly heal without love, connection, and deep caring would be delusion. We simply can't go the journey alone, especially if we're compromised by illness, injury, or emotional challenge. It is during these times that the support of others is never more critical. When we are at our lowest, we must allow grace to find us and open us for the flow of receiving. It is through experiencing other people showing up for you that you learn how to show up for others.

Learning how to do this can be a difficult part of the healing process. Many people can admit that they aren't very good at accepting help, and most of us want to do everything by ourselves. It's scary to lean on someone, especially when you're used to being the one who is leaned on. But, as Aretha Franklin said, "Ain't no way for me to love you, if you won't let me."

That's how it was for me, until my injury forced me to my knees. All of a sudden I couldn't work and with astronomical medical bills mounting, my family quickly stepped in to help; even insisting on paying my expenses. They were an absolute godsend. A beautiful array of friends swooped in to take care of the cooking, cleaning, laundry, and transportation to medical appointments. They showed up in ways that made me feel deeply love and valued, as did strangers once I began to get out and about more. On one occasion, a very kind gentleman noticed me struggling to get to my car with a bagful of groceries. He stopped and offered to carry my groceries the rest of the way. This is just one of several hundred examples of total strangers offering their love and support.

This was one of the biggest gifts in my healing process: learning how to lean into the flow of receiving. In many ways, my traumatic injury was one of the best experiences of my life. I learned so much, including one of the major ways I said no to life by choosing not to receive. I learned that people want to help, that people love to love. By receiving, you are allowing them that joy. You are letting people connect. You are letting people love you.

The important thing is that you don't get stuck in receiving-only mode forever.

You will know that you are making progress in your healing journey when you start to notice where and when you are able give back, and that the desire to give comes from a place of strength, not from a place of codependence or wanting to be liked. Knowing the difference can be especially difficult if you are a well-trained people pleaser, a "helper" who, like me and many others, has trouble letting go of the control that service creates. Pay attention to how the giving or the desire to give feels—is it paired with anxiety, or is it expansive? Is it rooted in fear or in love?

It's often the case that the universe will connect you with the right traveling companions at exactly the right time. Remember, the higher intelligence of life knows what you need and when. Remaining open to new connections will allow for grace to transpire in your life in the form of meaningful connections. I've had many amazing chance encounters when the universe put people in my life exactly when I was at a place where I could both genuinely give and receive. The relationships I formed were nourishing and sustainable—for both sides.

THE CALL OF THE SOUL AND THE STORY

Once you are feeling strong and stable, you can show up for others in ways that are impossible when you are ill or injured. Again, there's nothing wrong with taking more at times—all of us, at one point or another, will need more help than we can give. This is why, when we are strong, we must pay forward the love that others have given us. We'll need help again someday, and then we'll have the strength to give again, and then we'll need help, and so on in a cycle of giving and receiving.

When you are in a phase of strength, that is when it becomes possible for you to both reach new personal heights and reach beyond yourself. This is when it is essential for you to listen for those divine whispers—they will illuminate the next step in your journey. Now is the time to listen to the call of the soul.

What does the call of the soul feel like? The call of the soul can manifest in a wide range of amplitudes that vary from person to person. Some people receive more subtle, gentle signs, a sense of "rightness," while others feel a strong passion or fire. I suspect personality plays a role. Typically, those with calmer temperaments get softer messages; those with more exuberant, charismatic personalities experience their soul language as bigger and louder. Most of us experience both. Either way, each of our souls possesses deep intelligence that will communicate itself in the most effective way.

Regardless of where you fall on the amplitude spectrum, the call of the soul feels like an intense pull toward something, someone, or somewhere. There's an immense energetic force to it; a deep longing to move toward greater growth and healing. Listen intently, and do not let fear, doubt, or self-limiting beliefs derail you from following through on the call of the soul. Let go of the need to control, the need to logic your way through. It may be scary at first, like you are a baby bird peering over the edge of the nest for the first time. It may require you to leave the comfort of home in exchange for uncertainty, to let go of the *supposed-tos* and *shoulds* of conditioning in order to follow your own unique path. As Joseph Campbell said, If you can see your path laid out in front of you step by step, you know it's not your path. Your own path you make with every step you take, that's why it's your path."

Don't wait until the circumstances are perfect—they never will be. Don't wait until you are perfect—you will always have shadows. Embrace the fear and go.

You are leaving survival behind; you are beginning to thrive.

Now you can share your story. This isn't therapy or complaining or a request for help or attention—this is your hero's journey; how you survived, overcame, triumphed, and learned invaluable lessons along the way.

> *"Tell the story of the mountain you climbed. Your words could become a page in someone else's survival guide."—Morgan Harper Nichols*

It takes tremendous courage to share your story because it requires you to expose your vulnerability and to let go of your carefully designed persona and reveal the raw *unedited* version that includes all of you, including the quirky bits, the crazy sides, the regrets and the imperfections. Kinda scary, right? Absolutely. Most of us are very selective about the experiences we choose to share. We avoid sharing stories that make us feel vulnerable, ashamed, silly or arrogant, or we can't even fathom that anyone would be remotely interested.

But the benefits of sharing far outweigh the consequences of staying small and quiet. When we share our experiences, *we heal ourselves and we heal each other.* By sharing your story, you free yourself. By sharing your story, you find meaning in the most painful circumstances and a greater sense of purpose and direction in your life. By sharing your story, you allow others to connect with you in a genuine and beautiful way.

We become empowered by sharing our stories while lighting the way for those walking a similar path. In sharing your story, you will change the course of your life, and you may, in effect, change the course of someone else's life. There's a higher purpose to all you've been through. In sharing with others, you begin to breathe life into that very purpose. This is how you transform experience to insight to love. This is how you let others love you and give your love to the world. Because at the end of the day, we are all walking each other home.

Reflection Questions

I'd like to invite you to take a deep breath and answer the following questions as honestly as possible.

- Think about the people closest to you. Do these individuals and/or groups nourish you or deplete you?
- What are some old habits of relating that no longer align with your higher purpose? With whom in your life do you fall back into those habits?
- What are some new habits of relating you would like to develop? Who in your life has those habits?
- What is your relationship with social media? When is it healthy? When is it not healthy?
- How do you feel about setting boundaries? How do you feel about letting relationships go?
- How comfortable are you with receiving love? In what ways could you open yourself up to the flow of love?
- What is at the root of the care and support you give? Do you give out of fear or wanting to be liked, or out of a place of strength and love?
- What is the next step on your healing journey? Are you ready to share your story?

EPILOGUE

"You've seen my descent. Now watch my rising."
—Rumi

There is no redemption to this story, no happy ending or res-olution that ties my pain and heartache, resiliency and effort and awakening, into a tidy little bow. That's because life goes on until it doesn't, and my story is far from over. For the first few decades of my life, I kept my nose to the grindstone, never letting up no matter how worn down I got. Then my body, my life, said, *No. This is not all there is. You will stop—I will make you stop. Now. And you must find another way.*

No one wants pain. But when it arrives it brings a mes-sage. For a very long time, I didn't listen, didn't want to hear it. At a certain point, however, I had to admit that I was lost, and in that admission I humbled and opened myself to the universe. Slowly, painful step by painful step, I found my way back to myself, relearned the inner wisdom that had always existed within me, that always exists within each of us. I stopped fighting and started listening. I stopped fighting and started letting go.

What I've learned is that it's OK to fall. In those moments when the hurt seems insurmountable, it's OK to lie down and just breath. This is not giving up. This is giving yourself over to the ongoing river of change. If you allow it, it will take you in the direction of your soul's calling. Know that it'll be a ride full of twists, turns, and rapids—that's what makes it interesting. If life is always guiding us to where we need to be, then adversity is another step toward our highest self.

What I've learned is that it's OK to be confused. Pain has a way of making us feel separate from one another, to forget that we are all connected since time began and until time ends. It is also an opportunity to wake up, a pinch that shocks you out of the dream in which you've been living and into a reality that is not always pretty but has the potential to bring deeper clarity, a more expansive vision. If life is always guiding us to where we need to be, then we do not need to be afraid.

What I've learned is that it's OK to let go. I don't have the answers, and neither do you. Isn't that a comfort? You don't have to try so hard, to push away some things and grasp onto others. Instead, let the magnificent force, the divine, the universe unfold for you. As Lao Tzu said, "Water is fluid, soft, and yielding. But water will wear away rock, which is rigid and cannot yield. As a rule, whatever is fluid, soft, and yielding will overcome whatever is rigid and hard. This is another paradox: what is soft is strong." If life is always guiding us to where we need to be, then we don't need to fight life, especially at its most difficult or unpredictable. We can have the strength and the softness of water. We can relax into whatever life brings and relax into wherever life takes us.

Remember, life is always working for you, never against you. All you have to do is show up with curiosity, compassion, and a willingness to remind yourself that yesterday is over and tomorrow is an infinity of possibilities. You and only you have the power to change your life. But first, you must choose to do so and believe that you can.

I believe in you, and I wish you the best of luck and love on your lifelong process of transformation.

ENDNOTES

1   Daugherty, Greg. (March, 2012). Seven Famous People Who Missed the Titanic. *Smithsonian Magazine*, https://www.smithsonianmag.com/history/seven-famous-people-who-missed-the-titanic-101902418/.

2   WHO Guidelines on Hand Hygiene in Health Care: First Global Patient Safety Challenge Clean Care Is Safer Care. Geneva: World Health Organization; 2009. 4, Historical perspective on hand hygiene in health care. Available from: https://www.ncbi.nlm.nih.gov/books/NBK144018/

3   Nix, Elizabeth. (July, 2019). Tuskegee Experiment: The Infamous Syphilis Study. History, https://www.history.com/news/the-infamous-40-year-tuskegee-study.

4   Westervelt, Amy. (April, 2015). The medical research gap: how excluding women from clinical trials is hurting our health. The Guardian, https://www.theguardian.com/lifeandstyle/2015/apr/30/fda-clinical-trials-gender-gap-epa-nih-institute-of-medicine-cardiovascular-disease.

5   Fetters, Ashley. (August, 2018). The Doctor Doesn't Listen to Her. But the Media Is Starting To. *The Atlantic*, https://www.theatlantic.com/family/archive/2018/08/womens-health-care-gaslighting/567149/.

6   Villarosa, Linda. (April, 2018). Why America's Black Mothers and Babies Are in a Life-or-Death Crisis. *The New York Times Magazine*, https://www.nytimes.com/2018/04/11/magazine/black-mothers-babies-death-maternal-mortality.html.

7   U.S. Department of Health and Human Services. (September, 2020). What is the U.S. Opioid Epidemic?. https://www.hhs.gov/opioids/about-the-epidemic/index.html.

8   Hamlin, J. Kiley; Wynn, Karen; Bloom, Paul. (March, 2010).
     Three-month-olds show a negativity bias in their social evalua-
     tions. Developmental Science, volume 13 (6). https://
     onlinelibrary.wiley.com/doi/abs/10.1111/j.1467-7687
     .2010.00951.x

9   Goldsmith, K., & Dhar, R. (2013). Negativity bias and task moti-
     vation: Testing the effectiveness of positively versus negatively
     framed incentives. *Journal of Experimental Psychology: Applied,*
     19(4), 358–366. https://doi.org/10.1037/a0034415

10   Kiken, Laura G., & Shook, Natalie J. (2011). Looking Up:
     Mindfulness Increases Positive Judgments and Reduces Negativity
     Bias. *Social Psychological and Personality Science,* volume 2 (4),
     425-431. https://doi.org/10.1177/1948550610396585

11   Carstensen, Laura L., & DeLiema, Marguerite. (2017). The
     positivity effect: a negativity bias in youth fades with age.
     Behavioral Sciences, volume 19, 7-12. https://doi.org/10.1016/j
     .cobeha.2017.07.009

12   Sehgal, M, et al. (2013). Learning to learn —intrinsic plas-
     ticity as a metaplasticity mechanism for memory formation.
     Neurobiology of Learning and Memory, volume 105, 186-199.
     https://doi.org/10.1016/j.nlm.2013.07.008

13   Holt-Lunstad, J.; Smith, T.B.; Layton, J.B. (2010). Social
     Relationships and Mortality Risk: A Meta-analytic Review.
     PLoS Med 7(7): e1000316. https://doi.org/10.1371/journal.
     pmed.1000316

14   Berkman, L.F. & S.L. Syme. (1979). Social Networks, Host
     Resistance, and Mortality: A Nine-Year Follow-Up Study of
     Alameda County Residents. American Journal of Epidemiology,
     volume 109 (2), 186-204; T.A. Glass et al. (1999). Population-
     Based Study of Social and Productive Activities as Predictors
     of Survival Among Elderly Americans. British Medical Journal,
     volume 319 (728), 478-83; Wolf, S. & J.G. Bruhn. (1998).
     The Power of Clan: The Influence of Human Relationships on
     Heart Disease. (Piscataway, NW: Transaction Publishers);

Holahan, C.J. et al. (2010), Late-Life Alcohol Consumption and Twenty-Year Mortality. *Alcoholism, Clinical and Experimental Research*, volume 34 (11).